Antidepressants: The Practitioner's Guide

Dr. Shlomo Brook, M.D.

Copyright © 2014 Dr. Shlomo Brook

All rights reserved.

All rights reserved. No part of this book may be reproduced or transmitted in any form or any means, electronic or mechanical, including photocopying, recording or any information storage or retrieval system without permission from the copyright holder.

Although every effort has been made to ensure that all owners of copyright material have been acknowledged in this publication, I would be glad to acknowledge in subsequent reprints or editions any omissions brought to my attention. The information in this book has been compiled by way of general guidance in relation to the specific subjects addressed, but not a substitute and not to be relied on for medical, health care, pharmacological or other professional advice. Although every effort has been made to ensure that drug doses and another information is presented accurately, the ultimate responsibility rests with the prescribing physician. Neither the publishers nor the authors can be held responsible for errors or for any consequences arising from the use of information contained herein. Please consult your therapist before changing, stopping or starting any medical treatment. The author disclaims, in accordance with the law, any liability arising directly or indirectly from the use, or misuse of the information contained in this book.

ISBN-13: 978-1494979737

ISBN-10: 149497973X

Published by CreateSpace, First edition 2014

Copyright © 2014 Dr Shlomo Brook

brook@global.co.za

To my wife Justyna

CONTENTS

	Acknowledgments	i
1	Major Depression	Pg 10
2	Neurobiological basis of depression	Pg 22
3	The clinical use of antidepressants	Pg 37
4	Drug metabolism	Pg 52
5	Agomelatine	Pg 63
6	Bupropion	Pg 80
7	Citalopram	Pg 98
8	Chlomipramine	Pg 118
9	Desvenlafaxine	Pg 139
10	Duloxetine	Pg 154

11 Fluoxetine	Pg 177
12 Fluvoxamine	Pg 197
13 Imipramine	Pg 216
14 Milnacipran	Pg 235
15 Mirtazapine	Pg 255
16 Paroxetine	Pg 273
17 Sertraline	Pg 292
18 Tranylcypromine	Pg 312
19 Trazodone	Pg 334
20 Venlafaxine	Pg 353
21 Vilazodone	Pg 374
22 Vortioxetine	Pg 388

Preface

Depression is a common and debilitating condition, which affects approximately one in eight people in the US (1). In addition it is expected to be the second-leading cause of disability in the world by the year 2020 (2). Nearly 10% of all primary care office visits are related to depression (3). Untreated depression carries an increased risk of morbidity and mortality from general medical conditions (5). Medical care costs may significantly decreased in remitted patients. Patients recovered from depression have 49% lower medical costs in the year following their treatment compared with patients whose depression persisted (6).

Depression can be treated successfully and remission is the aim of depression treatment, as it is associated with a return of normal psychosocial function, lower rates of relapse, lower risk of suicide and alcohol or drug abuse, lack of disabling symptoms and overall a better prognosis (4). Unfortunately, up to 30% of the patients with major depression remain depressed after one year of treatment. I hope that this book will serve you as a useful guide for the treatment of your depressive patients.

Reference

1 RC Kessler, P Berglund, O Demler et al.: The epidemiology of MD: results from the national comorbiditysurvey replication (NCS-R). Jama 2003;289:3095-3105.

2 CJ Murray, AD Lopez. Global mortality, disability and the contribution of risk factors: Global burden of disease study. Lancet 1997;349:1436-1442.

3 RS Stafford, JC Ausiello, B Misra et al. national patterns of depression treatment in primary care. J Clin Psychiatry 2000; 2:211-216.

4 MH Trivedi, AJ Rush, SR Wisnieski et al. Evaluation of outcome with citalopram for depression. Am J Psychiatry 2006;163:28-40.

5 JM Zajecka. Treating depression to remission. J Clin Psychiatry 2003:64 (15):7-12.

6 GE Simon, D Reviki, J Heilitigenstein et al. Recovery from depression, work productivity, and health care costs among primary care patients. Gen Hosp Psychiatry 2000;22:153-162.

1
MAJOR DEPRESSION

Major depression is a mental disorder, that comprises emotional, cognitive and physical symptoms, all of which have a deleterious impact upon the patient's day-to-day functioning in various life areas such as work, relationships, academic pursuits and leisure activities.

Epidemiology of depression

The life time prevalence of depression shows a large variation from country to country. According to the World Health Organization (WHO) data published in 2004, the prevalence of depressive disorder varies from 3% in Japan, and up to 17% in the US and other Western European countries.

The number of people who will experience depression during their lifetime ranges between 8%-12%. Every day, 1454 US citizens out of 100.000 will experience depression.

Depression has two peaks. The first depressive episode is most likely to develop between the ages of 30-40. The second peak occurs between the ages of 50-60.

According to the WHO, by 2020, depressive disorder will be the second-leading cause of disability, only second to HIV/Aids (1).

The annual economic cost of depression on the US economy was estimated to be $86 billion per annum (2).

The US yearly cost breakdown of depression is illustrated in Figure 1.1

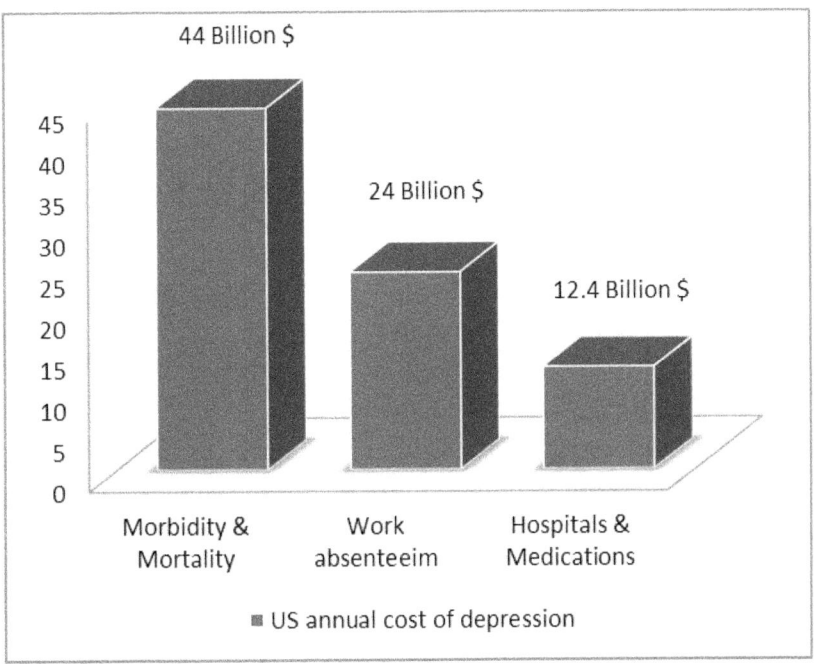

Figure 1.1 The annual cost of depression to the US economy. Adapted from PE Greenberg, SA Leon, HG Birnbaum. Cost of depression: Current assessment and future directions. Expert Rev Pharmaco- Economic Outcome Res 2001, 1:89-96.

Moreover, the indirect cost of depression due to increased use of social services, failure to reach maximum potential, job loss, disability and decreased productivity, further cripples the individual and the state economy.

Symptoms of depression

The symptoms of depression can be divided into three principal domains:

- The emotional domain
- The cognitive domain
- The physiological domain

The emotional domain

Depression is associated with severe emotional symptoms. The most prominent emotional symptoms of depression are low mood associated with a pervasive feeling of sadness, irritability, tension and anxiety.

The emotional symptoms of depression, tend to develop early at the onset of the illness and often fluctuate during the course of the day.

Some patients may feel much worse during the morning and improve as the day progresses, while others may experience a completely opposite emotional reaction with a reasonable emotional state in the morning and a severe depressive state at night.

The emotional depressive symptoms may have daily fluctuations with some positive days alternating with highly emotional depressive ones.

The cognitive domain

Depression is associated with severe cognitive symptoms. Cognition becomes negatively distorted. A pessimistic outlook on the past, the present and the future is highly prevalent. Memories become negatively tinted and any forthcoming events become bleak and frightening.

Any positive aspect of the past, the present and the future are completely ignored.

Thought of death and suicide become a frequent feature during the depressive state. Feelings of being a burden to the family and on the society become considerably prevalent while planning one's death may bring some relief. Suicide plans coupled with initial action are highly dangerous.

Patients exhibiting suicidal ideation and carrying out "planning" actions such as patients collecting medication for a planned overdose or writing a goodbye letter to their loved ones are at very high risk for suicide and require urgent antidepressant treatment and constant supervision, by a trained mental health professionals preferably on an in-patient psychiatric unit.

Reduced concentration is another disturbing yet highly common cognitive feature of depression. Initially, the patient may experience minor memory lapses usually interpreted as possible memory problems. However, reduced concentration may become a serious problem as it may interfere with work and home functionality.

In the severe depressive state, the patient may develop somatic and paranoid ideations. In such a circumstance, the patients may falsely believe of having a terminal illness or that somebody is planning to hurt them.

Patients can firmly believe that ordinary physical symptoms such as headache or back pain are symptoms of a terminal incurable cancer. Delusion of poverty is another serious psychotic interpretation of reality in which the patient may falsely believe of being financially broken. Such a break from reality may require hospitalization and intensive pharmacological treatment.

Loss of interest in personal and social activities is a common feature of depression. Depressed patients may experience reduced energy coupled with low self-esteem and lack of confidence in themselves. Feeling of inadequacy, in the presence of others, may result in social withdrawal and avoidance of a human company.

The physiological domain

The physiological symptoms of depression develop early during the illness. Depressed patients may experience sleep

difficulties, which include inability to fall asleep or inability to maintain sleep. Overall sleep time and sleep quality are severely reduced and may impact negatively on functioning the following day.

Energy levels become extremely low and are associated with feeling of tiredness. Appetite may be also affected during the depressive state with either an increase in, or, more frequently, decreased appetite with subsequent significant weight gain or weight loss. Food may become tasteless, and in severe cases, there is a total loss of appetite.

Sex drive is also affected during the depressive state and is experienced as reduces libido and inability to reach orgasm.

Most antidepressant medications aggravate the low sex drive and should be carefully addressed by the therapist.

The full range of the depressive symptom is illustrated in Figure 1.2

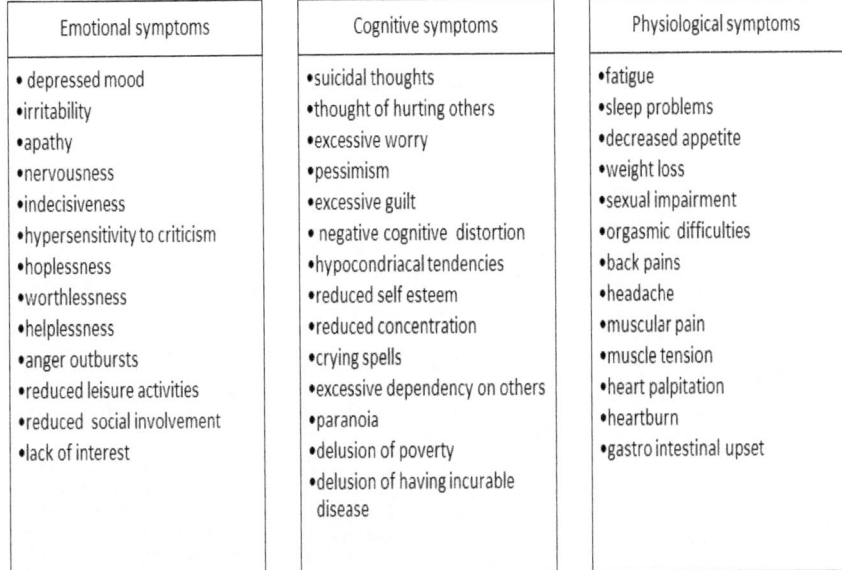

Figure 1.2: Depressive symptoms

The course of depression

Untreated depression can continue relentlessly and may become chronic. The average length of untreated depression is between six to nine months (3). Treatment of depression can take up to three months in order to achieve a full recovery.

Up to 25% of treated patients may experience the depressive episode longer then a year. It appears that 80% of patients with major depression will experience additional depressive episodes, which will follow the index episode.

On average, a depressed patient may experience up to five episodes (3).

The terminology of depression treatment responses

- **Response:** Response is defined as at least a 50% reduction in the depressive symptoms.

- **Remission:** Remission is defined as lack of depressive symptom, and is associated with return of normal psychosocial function.

- **Recovery:** Recovery refers to the period in which the patient is in a full remission and without depressive symptoms.

- **Relapse:** Relapse refers to the resumption of the depressive symptoms during the remission period.

- **Recurrence:** Recurrence refers to the onset of a new depressive episode which follows a period of recovery.

Major depression is associated with high levels of morbidity and mortality. The high mortality rates of depression result from suicide, which is twice of that of the general population as well as from accidents, cardiovascular disease and substance misuse (3). It appears that each new depressive episode increases the risk of chronicity.

In an uncomplicated depressive episode, 50% of the patients treated with a single antidepressant medication will experience a clinically significant improvement (4). However, only 20% - 35% of the patients will reach remission despite adequate pharmacological treatment (5).

Evidence from practice setting demonstrates that inadequate

antidepressant treatment is most likely to contribute to the low remission rates (7). Unfortunately, even successfully treated depressive patients can experience new relapses while on medications. Studies showed that the recurrence rates of depression, can reach up to 60% in the five years after treatment was stopped. However, with having more than two depressive episodes, the probability of getting a third depressive episode increase up to 70%. Depressed patient who have had three or more depressive episodes have a 90% probability to experience further episodes.

There is a large body of evidence to suggest that the longer the depressive state lasts, the more likely it is to persist (8). In addition, patients who did not recover from a depressive episode within the first two months of illness had only a one in three chance of recovery over the following two months (9). Furthermore, the steady decline in symptom improvement can reach merely a 7o% response rate in the second year in untreated depressive patients (9).

Chronic depression is a situation in which the depressive symptoms continue longer than two years regardless of treatment.

Follows is a list of the most common predictors to have a chronic depressive course (10):

- Having family history of depression.
- Presence of multiple losses.
- Presence of an additional chronic medical condition.
- Substance dependence.
- Unemployment.
- Having financial difficulties.

Early treatment discontinuation invariably results in relapse, which further highlights the importance of a prompt and optimal intervention. The factors that may predict future depressive recurrence can be divided into patient-related factors and illness-related factors.

The patient related-factors for future recurrence

- Family history of depression.
- Concomitant use of alcohol and or drugs.
- Thyroid abnormalities.
- Presence of chronic medical condition such as diabetes, hypothyroidism, Cushing syndrome.
- Chronic use of anti-hypertensive medication.
- Presence of high levels of stress.
- Death of a close relative or a friend.
- Divorce.
- Separation.
- Financial problems.
- Legal problems.

The illness-related factors for future recurrence

- Presence of a previous history of depression (each episode substantially increases the likelihood to develop another one).
- Having a current severe depressive episode.
- Presence of residual depressive symptoms.
- Getting the first episode after the age of 60 years.
- A seasonal pattern of depressed episodes.

For many years, remission was not a feasible goal in the treatment of depression due to side effects and safety-related issues of the old antidepressants. Patients and therapist accepted only partial symptomatic relief as a reasonable outcome despite the risk of relapse and recurrence (11).

The failure to achieve remission resulted in high morbidity and mortality, impaired psychosocial function and increase relapse rates. An additional consequence of failure to achieve remission was potential long-term treatment resistance (11).

Today, symptomatic remission and a return to premorbid social and occupational function has become the recommended goal for the management of depression (11).

With the introduction, in the 1980s, of the selective serotonin reuptake inhibitors (SSRIs) and later with the introduction of dual-action antidepressants, the drugs provided an improved safety and tolerability profile. This has resulted in more patients being able to achieve remission.

Despite the huge progress in recognition and treatment of depressive disorder, many patients with depression are still either not able to access these treatments or do not receive the optimal treatment for their mental condition resulting in an unnecessary suffering, increased morbidity and mortality, and reduced level of functioning.

The huge progress in recognition and treatment of depressive disorder, many patients with depression are still either not able to access these treatments or do not receive the optimal treatment for their mental condition resulting in an unnecessary suffering, increased morbidity and mortality, and reduced level of functioning.

Major depression references

1 Murray CJ, Lopez A.D. Global mortality, disability and the contribution of risk factors: Global burden of disease study. Lancet 1997;349:1436-1442

2 Greenberg PE, Leon S A, Birnbaum H G. Cost of depression: Current assessment and future directions. Expert Rev Pharmacoeconomic Outcome Res 2001, 1:89-96.

3 Gelder M, Mayaou R, Cowen P. Shorter Oxford Textbook of Psychiatry. Oxford University Press, 2001.

4 Gayness B N, Rush J, Wisnieski S R. The Star*D study: treating depression in the real world. Cleveland cli J of Medicine 2008 volume 75 :1:57-66.

5 Fava M, Davidson K G. Definition and epidemiology of treatment resistant depression. Psy Clin North Am 1996;19:179-200.

6 Regier D, Narrow W, Rae D et al. The de facto US mental and addictive disorder service system: epidemiologic catchment area prospective 1-year prevalence rates of disorders and services. Arch Gen Psychiatry 1993;50:85-94.

7 Trivedi MH, Rush AJ, Wisnieski SR et al. Evaluation of outcome with citalopram for depression. Am J Psychiatry 2006;163:28-40.

8 Piccinelli M, Wilkinson G. Outcome of depression in psychiatric setting. Br J Psychiatry, 1994;164:297-304.

9 Coryell W. Predictors of relapse into major depressive disorder in a non-clinical population. Am J Psychiatry 1991; 148:1353-1358.

10 Fochtman L J. Animal studies of ECT: Foundation for future research. Psychopharmacology Bull 1994;30:321-344.

11 Zajecka JM. Treating depression to remission. J Clin Psychiatry 2003:64 (15):7-12.

2

NEUROBIOLOGICAL BASIS OF DEPRESSION

The human brain consists of approximately 100 billion nerve cells, which are constantly interacting and communicating with each other through more than 40 recognized neurotransmitters.

The activation of the pre-synaptic neuron results in the release of small molecules synthesized from amino acids and stored in endoplasmatic vesicles. The released neurotransmitters into the synapse can either activate or inhibit their corresponding receptors by turning them on or off. The unused neurotransmitters are transported back into the presynaptic neurons via special reuptake transporters, specific to each biogenic amine.

Out of the 40 recognized neurotransmitters, there are three biogenic amines, which are putatively involved with depression. They are norepinephrine (NE), serotonin (5-HT) and dopamine (DA).

Norepinephrine (NE)

Norepinephrine is one of the most common neurotransmitter within the brain. The norepinephrine cell bodies are located within the brainstem and hypothalamus, and in an area called the locus ceruleus.

The locus ceruleus, located within the pons and is consists of cells containing norepinephrine. The locus ceruleus projects, principally to the prefrontal cortex as well as to the limbic system.

Norepinephrine metabolism is illustrated in Figure 2.1

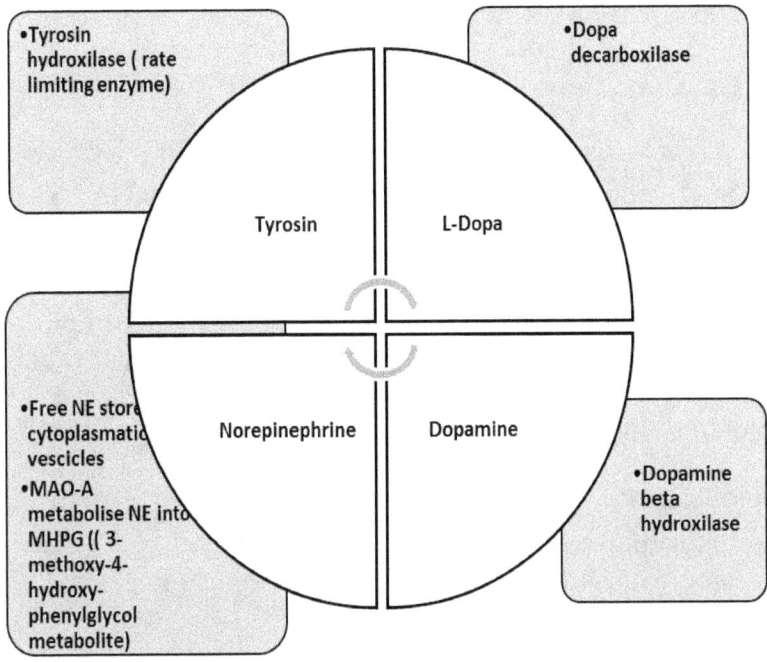

Figure 2.1: Norepinephrine metabolism

Norepinephrine is involved in the following brain functions:

- Attention
- Concentration
- Information processing
- Working memory
- Arousal state
- Wakefulness
- Emotions
- Energy feelings
- Fatigue
- Agitation

- Retardation

Serotonin (5-HT)

Serotonin was discovered in 1948 by researchers at the Cleveland clinic, and chemically it was identified as 5-hydroxytryptamine. The majority of the serotonin cell bodies are located in the raphe nucleus which is situated in the brainstem. From the raphe nucleus, the serotoninergic cells project to the hippocampus and to the prefrontal cortex.

Serotonin is involved in following brain functions:

- Sleep
- Appetite
- Body temperature
- Blood pressure
- Pain perception
- Nausea
- Emotions
- Anxiety
- Obsessions
- Compulsions
- Phobia

Serotonin metabolism is illustrated in Figure 2.2:

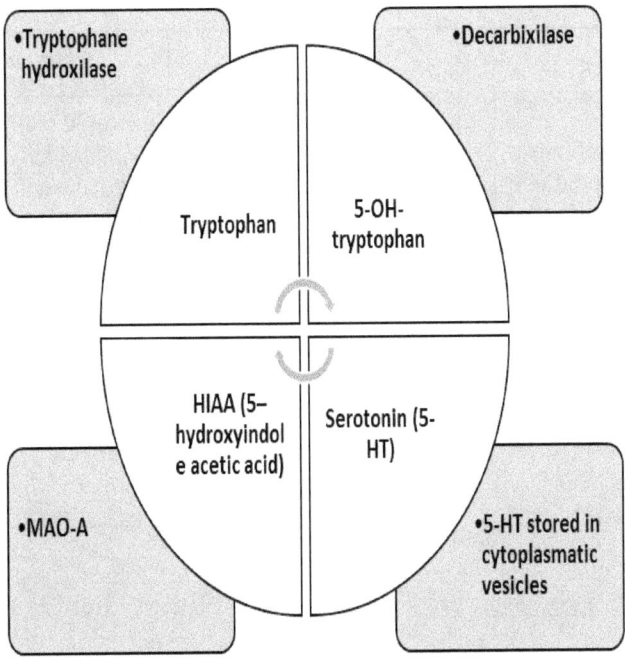

Figure 2.2: Serotonin metabolism

Today, there are at least nine identified serotonin receptors, which are located on the pre- and post-synaptic nerve cells. In addition, it appears that most serotonin receptors also have several subtypes.

The lists of pre-and post synaptic 5-HT receptors with their respective actions and possible involvement in psychological functioning are illustrated in the following figures 2.3 – 2.5

SERT	5HT1 B/D	5HT1A
• Reuptake transporter of free serotonin from the synaptic space back to the presynaptic nerve cell • **Possible involvement**: Depression • Anxiety • Cognition	• Detect the presence of free synaptic serotonin and block any further release of serotonin from the pre synaptic neuron. • **Possible involvement**: Depression • Anxiety • Cognition	• Located on the pre synaptic nerve cell. Its activation results in inhibition of the serotonin release to the synapse • **Possible involvement**: Depression • Anxiety • Cognition

Figure 2.3: <u>Pre- synaptic</u> 5-HT receptors and their respective actions

5-HT1A	5-HT2A	5-HT2C
• **Stimulate** the release of dopamine from the dopaminergic neurons. • Possible involvement: Depression • Anxiety • Hormone release • Cognition	• **Blocks** the release of dopamine from the dopaminergic neurons. • **Possible involvement**: Sleep • Hallucinations • Activate the movement related nerve cells	• **Regulates** the release of dopamine and norepinephrine from the cortex. • **Possible involvement**: Emotions • Weight • Cognition • Memory • Concentration • Attention

Figure 2.4 <u>Post- synaptic</u> 5-HT receptors and their respective actions

5-HT3	5-HT6	5-HT7
• **Blocks** the action of inhibitory interneurons. • **Possible involvement**: Nausea • Vomiting • Cognitive enhancement	• **Regulates** the release of brain derived neurotrophic factor (BDNF). • Possible involvement; Improve memory • Improve cell resilience • Improve nerve cell growth	• **Regulates** the circadian rhythms. • **Possible involvement**: Sleep • Emotions

Figure 2.5 <u>Post- synaptic</u> 5-HT receptors and their respective actions

Dopamine (DA)

Dopamine is another principal neurotransmitter involved with depression. Dopamine cell bodies are located in several brain areas with the following main projections:

- **Nigrostriatal projection**: The nigrostriatal pathway projects from the substantia nigra to the basal nuclei. This pathway is involved in coordination of motor functions.

- **Mesolimbic projections**: The mesolimbic pathway projects from the ventral tegmentum to the nucleus accumbens. This pathway is involved in reward and pleasure.

- **Mesocortical projections**: The mesocortical pathway projects from the ventral tegmentum to the frontal cortex and to the limbic cortex. This pathway is involved in emotions, pleasure, drive and reward.

- **Tuberoinfundibular projections:** The tuberoinfundibular pathway projects from the hypothalamus to the anterior pituitary gland. This pathway is involved in hormonal secretion.

The dopamine metabolism is illustrated in the following Figure 2.6

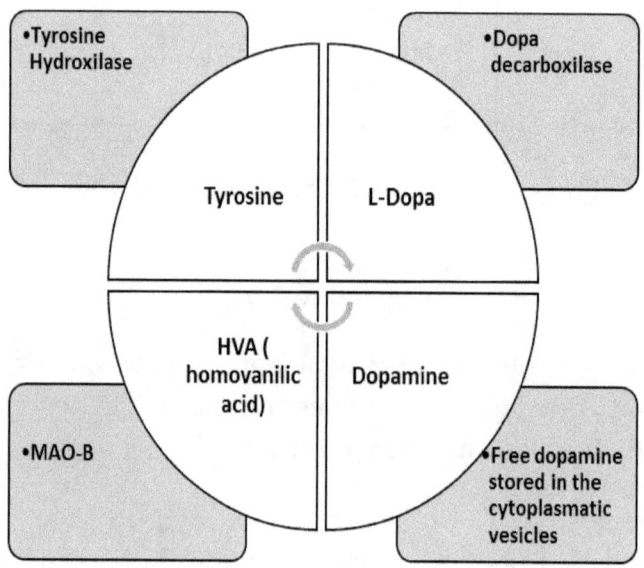

Figure 2.6: Dopamine metabolism

Historical overview of antidepressants

Since the late 1950s, the treatment of major depressive disorder (MDD) with antidepressants gained momentum and replaced other treatment modalities such as Freudian psychoanalysis, which had previously dominated the psychiatric management of MDD.

The increase knowledge of neuroanatomy, neurophysiology and neuro-pharmacology along with the advances in drug development and manufacturing led to a boom in the development of new antidepressants.

Imipramine was the first Tricyclic Antidepressant (TCA) to be developed. Imipramine was presented at the first International Congress of Neuropharmacology held in Rome in September 1958. Imipramine showed encouraging results in the treatment of 46 patients with depressive psychosis.

During the same period, several reports in the medical literature emerged, suggesting that an anti- tuberculosis agent called iproniazid was shown to have mood elevating properties.

Soon after, a number of drugs inhibiting the monoamine oxidase enzymes (MAO inhibitors, or MAOI) were developed and investigated for possible antidepressant efficacy.

The TCAs and MAOI antidepressants showed good antidepressant efficacy.

The antidepressant effects were related to their ability to block the norepinephrine and serotonin re-uptake transporters (in the case of TCAs), and to irreversibly block the MAO enzyme (MAO inhibitors), which resulted in increased levels of serotonin and norepinephrine in the brain.

For 30 years, the MAOIs and TCAs dominated the antidepressant markets despite having serious tolerability and safety issues which will be thoroughly discussed in the relevant chapters.

Nevertheless, over the years, the TCAs and MAOIs were reasonably effective in treating depression. However, their severe side effects seriously affected patient's adherence to treatment.

Many patients were unable to continue with the recommended treatment with TCA and MAOI and either terminated early the proposed treatment regimens or used sub-therapeutic doses.

The need to develop new antidepressants with improved tolerability and improved efficacy resulted in the development of the SSRIs which were introduced into the market in the mid-1980s.

The newly developed SSRIs gained enormous popularity due to their simplified use (once-a-day dose), better tolerability and improved safety with overdose, and yet with comparable efficacy to the older TCAs.

However, despite reasonable efficacy and improved tolerability, the severe sexual-related side effects that developed with the SSRIs, as well as the need for an at least 2-week waiting period before any treatment response, resulted in the necessity of development of alternative antidepressants.

During the 1990s, new antidepressants were introduced into the market with the promise of having better tolerability, safety in overdose and faster antidepressant action.

The Serotonin Norepinephrine Reuptake Inhibitors (SNRI) had dual action on the serotonin reuptake transporters as well as on the norepinephrine re uptake transporters. They provided some hope for faster and better antidepressant efficacy combined with improved tolerability.

However, that the SNRIs had better and faster efficacies was somewhat due to marketing success rather than actual clinical proof. Thus, the search for better and faster antidepressant continued.

Along came bupropion capable of inhibiting the dopamine

reuptake transporters (DAT), and agomelatine, the first antidepressant to inhibit melatonin receptors (with effects on the 5-HT2C receptors and the circadian rhythms).

However, despite brilliant marketing, even these new antidepressants had severe side effects and similar efficacy to that of the older antidepressants. This is where antidepressant medications stand today. Given that the array of drugs is still unsatisfactory, the search for improved antidepressant medications continues.

It appears that future research is moving beyond the Serotonin Reuptake Transporters (SERT), the Norepinephrine Reuptake Transporters (NET) and the Dopamine Reuptake Transporters (DAT) and towards targeting the post-synaptic serotonin receptors located on the serotoninergic neurons in the amygdala and in the limbic system.

The current focus of research is on the post-synaptic 5-HT1A – agonists, 5 –HT 2A antagonists, 5-HT2C antagonists and 5 –HT 1D antagonists.

These newly targeted receptors appear to be involved with depressive mood, anxiety, insomnia and agitation and may produce a more potent and faster response, along with an improved tolerability and safety profile.

The hope is that the new medications will have quicker onset and safer action, which will ultimately improve adherence to treatment and will consequently improve remission rates and functionality of depressed patients.

Categories of antidepressants

TCAs

The TCAs are antidepressants, that were developed in 1957 after the discovery by the Swiss psychiatrists, Roland Kuhn, of the calming effects of imipramine on agitated depressed patients. All the TCAs have a basic three-ring structure, and all have a broad range of receptor affinity, which is responsible for their low tolerability and poor safety in overdose and can be lethal in overdose.

In addition, the TCAs have a strong affinity for the adrenergic α1, histaminergic H1, and acetylcoline Ach receptors, which results in their strong anticholinergic side effect profile. These anticholinergic symptoms include dry mouth, blurred vision, constipation, and urinary retention as well as excessive sedation, weight gain and hypotension.

Figure 2.7 reflects the affinity of TCAs for the 5-HT, NE, DA, α1, H1 and Ach receptors with their effective clinical doses.

Imipramine	Clomipramine	Amitriptyline
• 5-HT +++	• 5-HT++++	• 5-HT +
• NE +++	• NE +++	• NE++++
• DA +	• DA +	• DA+
• α1+++	• α1+++	• α1+++
• H1+++	• H1 +++	• H1++++
• ACh+++	• ACh +++	• ACh ++
• Dose range: 75-300mg	• Dose range: 25-250mg	• Dose range: 50-300mg

Figure 2.7: TCAs receptor affinity spectrum. Key: + = minimal, ++ = mild, +++ = moderate, ++++ = strong, +++++ = very strong.

Maprotiline	Amoxapine	Lofepramine
• 5-HT +	• 5-HT ++	• 5-HT ++
• NE ++++	• NE ++++	• NE ++++
• DA +	• DA +	• DA +
• α1 +++	• α1 +++	• α1 ++
• H1 ++++	• H1 +++	• H1 ++
• ACh ++	• ACh ++	• ACh ++
• Dose range: 75-225	• Dose range: 50-600mg	• Dose range: 7--140mg

Figure 2.8: TCAs receptor affinity spectrum. Key: + = minimal, ++ = mild, +++ = moderate, ++++= strong, +++++ = very strong.

SSRI (Selective Serotonin Reuptake Inhibitors)

The SSRIs were developed in the early 1980s. The class currently includes five members who share a similar inhibitory effect on the serotonin reuptake transporter (SERT). Follows is a list of the serotonin reuptake transporter inhibitors according to their affinity to SERT.

- Paroxetine   (Highest affinity)
- Citalopram
- Fluvoxamine
- Sertraline
- Fluoxetine   (Lowest affinity)

Over the past year two additional antidepressant joined the market: Vilazodone in 2011 and Vortioxetine in 2013. Both newest member of the SSRI family show to have similar effect on SERT and on other 5-HT receptors.

Due to the lack of a direct correlation between the SSRIs plasma levels with their antidepressant effects, the SSRI antidepressant response rate is unaffected by daily dose increases. This results in a flat dose response curve. The lack of a dose response may be related to the SSRI's ability to block at least 80% of the serotonin re-uptake transporters at the lowest dose which has an antidepressant effect.

In addition to the inhibitory effect on SERT, all SSRIs are capable of blocking the 5-HT1A auto receptor which is situated on the pre synaptic nerve cell. These receptors have an on/off function for the production and the release of serotonin from the pre synaptic nerve cell.

Blocking the pre synaptic 5-HT1A receptors will enhance the production and the release of serotonin from the pre synaptic nerve cell, while the activation of the pre synaptic 5-HT1A receptors will significantly reduce the amount of serotonin released by the pre synaptic nerve cell.

Most SSRIs have a milder side effect profile compared to the older TCAs generation. Furthermore, it appears that most SSRIs produce an array of side effects which seems to be slightly more tolerable than those seen with the TCAs.

The most common side effects of the SSRIs class include anxiety and agitation, headache, nausea, gastrointestinal discomfort, increased bowel motility, GI cramps and diarrhea. The SSRIs also have strong sexual side effects, which include reduced sex drive, anorgasmia and delayed ejaculation.

The SSRIs sexual-related side effects are very common and affect at least a one-third of treated patients and will often reduce a patient's adherence to treatment. Fortunately, most of the SSRIs side effects are temporary and often tend to reduce over time.

Serotonin & Norepinephrine Reuptake Inhibitors: (SNRIs)

The SNRI class is a relatively new addition to the antidepressant family. The SNRIs have a strong affinity for both the serotonin and the norepinephrine reuptake transporters. The first SNRI agent to gain FDA approval for the treatment of major depression was venlafaxine. Several years later, three additional agents gained access to the antidepressant market.

The SNRI timeline is as follows:

- 1993 Venlafaxine
- 2004 Duloxetine
- 2008 Desvenlafaxine
- 2009 Milnacipram (Not approved by the FDA)

The SNRIs gained popularity amongst prescribers due to their proven antidepressant efficacy, good tolerability and relative safety in overdose.

Most SNRIs have an ability to inhibit the serotonin reuptake transporters (SERT) as well as the norepinephrine reuptake transporters (NET). This dual effect on SERT and NET may be responsible for the better antidepressant efficacy.

It appears that the current clinical data suggests that the SNRIs have a higher remission rate compared to the SSRIs. Moreover, venlafaxine seems to have better efficacy at higher doses, which is probably due to its ability to block both the serotonin and the norepinephrine reuptake transporters as well as the dopamine re uptake transporters (DAT).

It is speculated that the ability of the SNRIs to increase brain dopamine levels is more prominent in the prefrontal cortex, which is one of the key areas involved with mood.

3

The clinical use of antidepressants

Over the past 50 years, antidepressants have become the principal treatment modality for moderate to severe depression. Furthermore, currently there is sufficient evidence to suggest that long-term use of antidepressants can significantly reduce the risk of recurrence, as well as improve the patient's quality of life and their level of functioning.

All currently available antidepressants have an average of 60% response rate after the treatment of depression. In addition, all antidepressants require at least one to three weeks of continuous use to demonstrate a response.

The British National Clinical Practice Guidelines (NICE guidelines) published in 2004 suggest that SSRIs should be the first-line of treatment for depression because they are as effective as TCAs, and their use is less likely to be discontinued due to their favorable side-effect profile (1).

However, data from 93 trials of dual-action antidepressants, suggests that the newer-generation antidepressants have a possible better response rate of 63% compared to the older SSRIs class which have a response rate of 59% (2,3).

A study conducted in 2009 by Cipriani et al, found that the response rates to mirtazapine, escitalopram, venlafaxine and sertraline were superior to that of duloxetine, fluoxetine, fluvoxamine and paroxetine(4). However, sertraline, escitalopram and bupropion were, to a greater degree, better tolerated and more accepted by the patients than the rest of the antidepressants (4).

Residual symptoms of depression can predict recurrence (5). Follow-up studies with recovered patients found that 85% had a recurrence within 15 years (6). However, most studies showed that long-term use of antidepressants appear to prevent relapse (7).

Treatment strategies

Figure 3.1 shows a systematic strategy for the treatment of MDD

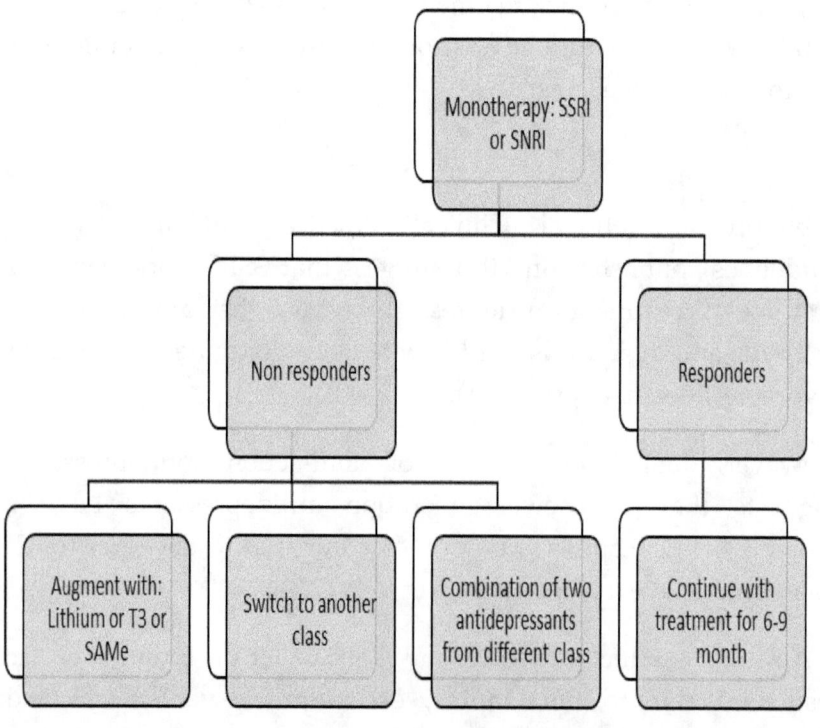

Figure 3.1: Antidepressant treatment strategies

Augmentation strategies

Lithium

In a Multicentre double – blind randomized parallel group clinical trial on the efficacy of the combination of clomipramine 150mg/day plus lithium carbonate 750mg/day versus clomipramine 150mg/day plus placebo for the treatment of unipolar MDD, the patients with lithium augmentation showed a significant improvement of the depressive symptoms within the first week of treatment (8). In this study, 79% of the patients who received lithium augmentation responded to the combined lithium and clomipramine treatment while 71% of the patients on clomipramine and placebo responded. Such optimistic results were not replicated in the STAR*D study which was conducted in the US and published in 2008. The STAR*D study enrolled 4,041 nonpsychotic depressed outpatients at 23 psychiatric and 18 primary care sites. 2786 patients were randomized and received citalopram for 12-weeks.

After 12-weeks of treatment, non responders were given either a different antidepressant or continued with citalopram augmented with bupropion or buspirone. Those patients who failed to respond were either switched to mirtazapine or placed subsequently, on Lithium carbonate augmentation or T3 augmentation (17).

The results of the STAR*D study showed that the augmentation with Lithium produced modest increase in response rates (9).

STAR*D Study design is illustrated in Figure 3.2

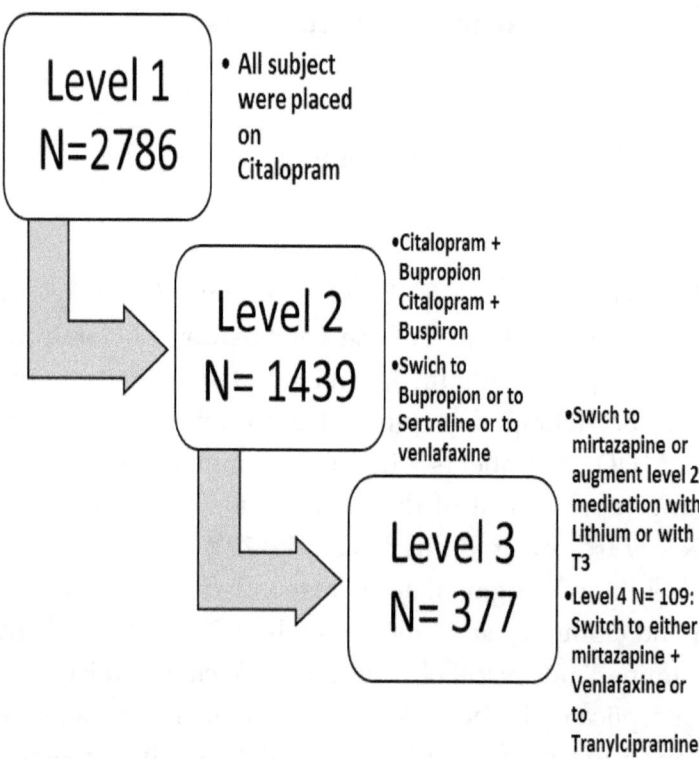

Figure 3.2 STAR*D study design

Thyroid Hormone (T3) augmentation

Early studies with Triiodothyronine (T3) showed some promise when it could improve depressive symptoms when augmented with antidepressants. However, in the STAR*D study the augmentation with T3 produced only a modest additional response rate (9). It appears that T3 is not likely to accelerate the clinical response to SSRIs in Major Depression (10).

SAMe

S-Adenosyl methionine (SAMe) was discovered in Italy by G.L Cantoni in 1952. SAMe is made from ATP and methionine and it is involved in numerous intracellular metabolic reactions as well as in cellular growth and repair.

SAMe is also involved in the biosynthesis of hormones and neurotransmitters, such as dopamine and serotonin.

SAMe is sold as a dietary supplement in a form of enteric-coated tablets. SAMe peak plasma concentration is reached in 3-5 hours and it has a half-life of 2 hours.

Early studies with S-adenosyl methionine (SAMe) showed some antidepressant promise, which led to consideration of its use as an augmentation to antidepressant medications. However, further studies are needed to explore the role of SAMe as an augmentation to antidepressant treatment.

Folic acid

Folic acid is the water soluble form of vitamin B9 and is essential for numerous bodily functions, such as DNA synthesis and repair, cell division and growth. Leafy vegetables are the principal source of folic acid as humans are not able to synthesize folic acid. Dietary low intake of Vitamin B9 may lead to folic acid deficiency which in developing embryos may result in neural tube defects while in adult it may cause macrocytic anemia peripheral neuropathy depression and cognitive impairment.

A recent study with 500mcg of folic acid augmentation to fluoxetine reported a 93% response rate, compared to only a 61%

response rate in patients who were treated with fluoxetine alone (11).

Lamotrigine

Several small studies with lamotrigine augmentation showed some modest improvement in depressed patient's response rates when compared to placebo augmentation of antidepressants.

In a small double-blind randomized placebo-controlled trial of augmentation with lamotrigine 100mg or placebo in patients concomitantly treated with fluoxetine for resistant MDD, the lamotrigine augmented group showed statistical superiority to placebo on the Clinical Global Impression (CGI) Scale scores (12).

However, the benefit of using anticonvulsants as augmentation to antidepressants as first-line treatment for MDD is still questionable (13).

Atypical antipsychotics

A meta- analysis of randomized controlled trials with atypical antipsychotic augmentation in patients with MDD found that such augmentation was significantly more effective than placebo. Further, there were no differences in efficacy between olanzapine, risperidone, quetiapine or aripiprazole augmentation (14).

However, the augmentation with atypical antipsychotics was associated with higher discontinuation rates due to side effects. These included weight gain and metabolic syndrome, over sedation, fatigue, somnolence, hyperprolactinemia, and dyslipidemia as well as extrapyramidal side effects, including akathisia, dystonic reactions, Parkinsonism and tardive dyskinesia

(13). In addition to safety and tolerability issues related to the atypical antipsychotic augmentation, the significant increase of cost merits additional consideration (2).

Antidepressant combination

It appears that the combination of two antidepressants with a different mode of action may increase the patient's response rates.

In a small double blind randomized study of antidepressant combination for the treatment of MDD (15), the combination of mirtazepine with fluoxetine, venlafaxine or bupropion was shown to produce statistically better remission rates than that of fluoxetine monotherapy. The results of this study are shown in figure 3.3

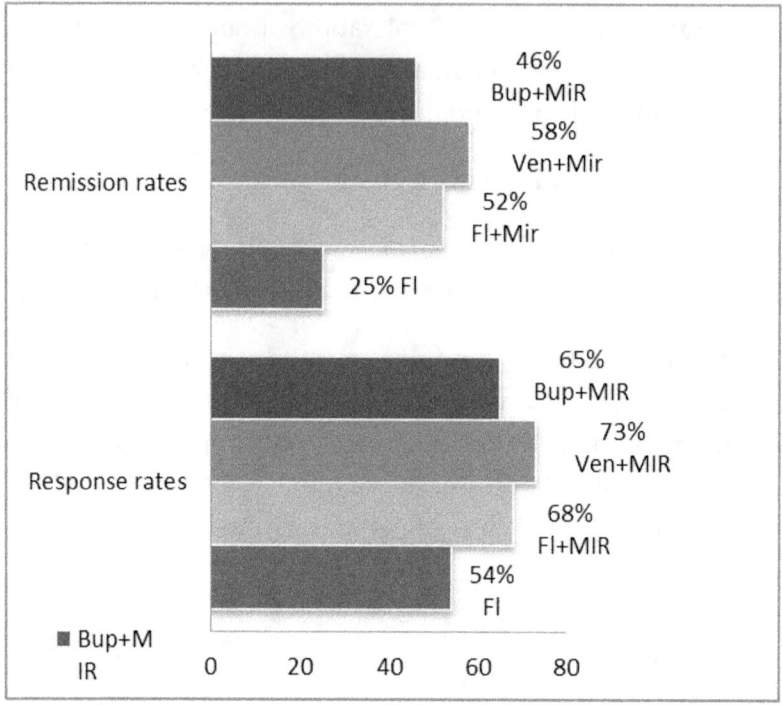

Figure 3.3 The various combination of mirtazapine (MIR), venlafaxine (VEN) or Bupropion (BUP) compared to fluoxetine (FL) monotherapy. Adapted from Blier P, Ward HE, Tremblay P et al. Combination of antidepressant medications from treatment initiation for MDD: a double blind randomized study. American Journal of Psychiatry. 2010, 167(3), 281-288.

The combination of antidepressants with different mode of action, particularly for the treatment resistant depressive patient may improve their response and remission rates. However, In addition to safety and tolerability issues related to the combination of two antidepressant medications, the significant increase in cost is an important consideration.

Modafinil

Modafinil is an agent approved by the FDA for the treatment of narcolepsy and shift work sleep disorder and as adjunctive treatment for obstructive sleep apnea syndrome. In a small randomized double-blind study (16), modafinil was added to SSRIs from the onset of treatment of MDD patients who also had fatigue and sleepiness. However, the combination of modafinil with SSRI did not show any significant improvement in the depressive symptoms over the group of patients treated only with SSRI.

Ketamine

Ketamine is a well know anesthetic widely used by anesthesiologist for sleep induction. Upon its administration, it is rapidly metabolized in the liver by microsomal enzymes into several metabolites. The *hydroxynorketamine* , is one of the principal metabolite of ketamine, increases the levels of the activating phosphorylated form of mammalian target of rapamycin (mTOR): a protein kinase involved in protein synthesis, synaptic plasticity and neurotrophic signaling. In addition, the mTOR inhibit the α7subtype of the nicotinic acetylcholine α7nACh receptors. It is possible that the ketamine induced antidepressants effects result by the rapid activation of the mTOR pathway in the prefrontal cortex with subsequent increase of multiple synaptic signaling proteins, dendrites density (synaptogenesis) and synaptic activity which results in behavioral responses indicative of mood improvement.

In a study published by Berman (18) in a nine patients with major depression, ketamine 0.5mg/kg was infused slowly over 40 minutes, produced rapid mood improvement that peaked after 72 hours.

Currently, ketamine is used only for a restricted number of

therapy-resistant-depressive cases and it is only used with a close cooperation with anesthesiologist.

Antidepressant use during pregnancy

Women with a history of mood disorder appear to be at risk for recurrence of depression during pregnancy, especially when antidepressants have been discontinued. Treatment of depression during pregnancy is related to the severity of illness, the past treatment response and the patient preferences.

The information regarding the effects of antidepressants when are used during pregnancy is incomplete. The risks of antidepressant use during pregnancy must be weight against the risks associated with untreated depression.

In general there are several risks to consider with the use of antidepressants during pregnancy:

- Risk of organ malformation (teratogenesis)
- Risk of miscarriage
- Risk of neonatal toxicity (withdrwal symptoms)
- Risk of neonatal development of Persistant Pulmonary Hypertension of the Newborn (PPHN)
- Risk of long- term neurobehavioural effects of the child.
- Risk of suicide in the untreated pregnant women
- Risk of development of Post Partum Depression

The FDA established a classification system based on data derived from human and animal studies. According the FDA classification, all antidepressants are classified into 5 risk categories A,B,C,D, and X.

Medications in category A are safe for use during pregnancy, whereas category X drugs are contraindicated due to their known potential to cause damage to the fetus.

Most antidepressants are classified as category C except some Tricyclic antidepressants and paroxetine which have been labeled as category D indicating positive evidence of risk. First trimester exposure to paroxetine was associated with an increased risk of cardiac defects.

At present the data regarding the use of SSRI and SNRI are still limited however, given the frequency of use of these medications during pregnancy, the data supporting their safety is increasing.

The risk of PPHN with SSRI after 20 weeks of pregnancy is in the range of 1%. However, the current data failed to demonstrate any association between SSRI use during pregnancy and PPHN.

A limited data is available on the long term effects of in-utero antidepressant exposure. Currently there is no evidence of cognitive development impairment, temperament, mood distractibility and activity level among children when followed through early childhood (19). Therefore, despite the reassuring data, further investigation into the long term effects of prenatal exposure to antidepressants is required.

In the less severe cases of depression, discontinuation of antidepressants therapy during pregnancy should be considered and the use of Cognitive Behavioural Therapy (CBT) should be used in order to reduce the risk of recurrence of depression during pregnancy.

Women who stopped their antidepressants, during pregnancy, were 5 times more likely to relapse, further emphasis the need to consider antidepressant use during pregnancy in high relapse risk group (20).

Women using antidepressants during their pregnancy should discontinue their antidepressant just before delivery to minimize the risk of neonatal toxicity which may develop in the neonate. The toxicity symptoms in the neonate include transient jitteriness, tachypnea and tremulousness. Unfortunately such strategy may increase the risk of depression in women entering the post-partum period.

Depressed women, who opted to continue with an antidepressant during pregnancy, experience high relapse rate. Up to 26% of the women on antidepressant experienced a relapse of major depression during pregnancy despite using antidepressants (20).

In cases of severe depression with suicidal behavior or psychotic symptoms, hospitalization should be considered and treatment with Electroconvulsive Therapy (ECT) may be selected. The use of ECT during pregnancy is relatively safe and highly efficacious (21).

Neurobiological basis of depression & antidepressant overview references

1 Nice guidelines 2004. Depression: Management of depression in primary and secondary care. National Clinical Practice Guidelines. Number 23. London: National Institute for clinical Excellence.

2 Stein D, Lerer B, Stahl SM: Essential Evidence – Based Psychopharmacology. Second edition. Cambridge University Press 2012.

3 Papakostas GI, Thase ME, Fava M et al: Are antidepressant drugs that combine serotonergic and noradrenergic mechanisms of action more effective than the SSRIs in treating MDD? A meta-analysis of studies of newer agents. Biological Psychiatry 2007;62:1217-1227.

4 Cipriani A, Furukawa TA, Salanti G et al. Comparative efficacy and acceptability of 12 new generation antidepressants: A multiple –treatment meta-analysis. Lancet 2009;373, 746-758.

5 Judd L, Akiskal HS, Maser JD et al. A prospective 12-years study of subsyndromal and syndromal depressive symptoms in unipolar MDD. J of Affective Disorder. 1998;50,97-108.

6 Mueller T, Leon AC, Keller MB et al. Recurrence after recovery from MDD during 15 years of observational follow up. American Journal of Psychiatry 1999,156;1000-1006.

7 Weiths KL, Houser T, Bately SR et al. Continuation phase treatment with bupropion SR effectively decreases the risk for relapse of depression. Biological Psychiatry. 2002, 51; 753-761.

8 Januel D, Poirier MF, D'alche-Biree F et al. Multicenter double – blind randomized parallel group clinical trial of efficacy of the combination clomipramine 150mg/day plus lithium 750mg/day versus clomipramine plus placebo in the treatment of unipolar MDD. Journal of Affective Disorder 2003;76(1-3), 191-200.

9 Rush AJ, Trivedi MH, Wisniewski SR et al. Acute and longer term outcomes in depressed outpatients requiring one or several treatment steps: A STAR*D report. American Journal of Psychiatry 2006, 163, 1905- 1917.

10 Papakostas GL, Cooper-Kazaz R, Appelhof BC et al. Simultaneous initiation of pharmacotherapy with T3 and SSRI for MDD. A quantitative synthesis of double-blind studies. International Clinical Psychopharmacology. 2009, 24(1), 19-25.

11 Coopen A Bailey J. Enhancement of the antidepressant action of fluoxetine by folic acid: A randomized, placebo controlled trial. Journal of Affective Disorders. 2000, 60(2), 121-130.

12 Barbosa L, Berk M, Voster M. A double-blind randomized placebo-controlled trial of augmentation with lamotrigine or placebo in patients concomitantly treated with fluoxetine for resistant MDD. Journal of Clinical Psychiatry 2003. 64, 403-407.

13. Papakostas GI, Fava M. Pharmacotherapy for depression and treatment resistant depression. World Scientific 2010.

14 Nelson JC, Papakostas GI. Atypical antipsychotic augmentation in MDD: A meta analysis of placebo-controlled randomized trials. American Journal of Psychiatry. 2009, 166, 980-991.

15 Blier P, Ward HE, Tremblay P et al. Combination of antidepressant medications from treatment initiation for MDD: a double blind randomized study. American Journal of Psychiatry. 2010, 167(3), 281-288.

16 Dunlop BW, Crits-Christoph P, Evans DL, et al. Co administration of modafinil and a SSRI from the initiation of treatment of MDD with fatigue and sleepiness: A double-blind, placebo controlled study. Journal of Clinical Psychopharmacology, 2007, 27(6), 614-619.

17 Warden D, Rush AJ, Trivedi Mh et al. The STAR*D Project results: A comprehensive review of findings. Curr. Psychiatry Rep. 2007, 9(6), 449-459.

18 Berman RM, Cappiello A, Anand A, Oren DA et al. Antidepressant effects of ketamine in depressed patients. Biol Psychiatry 2000;47;351-4

19 Nulman I, Rovert J, Stewart D et al: Neurodevelopment of children exposed in utero to antidepressant drugs, N Engl J Med 336:258-262,1997.

20 Cohen LS, Altshuler LL, Harlow BL, et al: Relapse of major depression during pregnancy in women who maintain or

discontinue antidepressant treatment. JAMA 295(5):499-507, 2006.

21 Anderson EL, Reti IM: ECT in pregnancy: a review of the literature from 1941 to 2007, Psychosom Med 71(2): 235-242, 2009.

4

Drug metabolism

The most common way by which the body metabolizes any administered drug is by biotransformation of the original compounds into either active or inactive metabolite.

The biotransformation process is mediated by enzymes located within the stomach, intestine, blood plasma, liver, kidney and in the brain. The liver is by far the most active site of drug biotransformation.

The most common liver enzymatic alteration of psycho active medications is oxidation, which transform the drug into a less lipid-soluble state thus reducing its ability to penetrate the blood-brain barrier.

Another form of hepatic biotransformation of psycho-active drug is the addition of glucuronide and sulphate, which render the original drug inactive and more water-soluble so that they can be excrete more efficiently by the kidneys.

Some psycho-active drugs are metabolized into active compounds, which also have antidepressant properties and may extend the action of the parent drug.

The hepatic enzymes are microsomal and lack specificity, thus are able to metabolize a wide range of ingested compounds. Among the most important microsomal liver enzymes are the cytochrome P450 (CYP) enzymes.

Cytochrome P450

To date, more than 30 members of the cytochrome P450 enzyme were identified, responsible for the metabolism of the majority of the psychiatric drugs as well as capable of detoxify multiple other foreign substances.

The first metabolic step of the CYP 450 enzymes is to convert the parent drug into a more polar compound in order to facilitate its excretion from the kidneys. The polarization of the parent compound occurs by either a process of oxidation, hydrolization or reduction and thereafter, the new metabolite is conjugated with sulphate or glucuronic acid in order to facilitate its excretion by the kidneys.

Some psycho-active drugs can induce the CYP enzymes either by increasing the enzyme production or by enhancing its activity. Carbamazepine is a CYP 450 3A4 inducer, which results in enhancement of its own metabolism and consequently resulting in a lower carbamazepine blood level.

Some psycho-active drugs are capable of inhibiting the activity of the CYP enzyme, which will reduce the enzyme metabolic efficiency. Examples of enzyme inhibitors are duloxetine and fluoxetine, which inhibit the activity of CYP 2D6 enzymes.

The inhibition of the 2D6 activity may interfere with the metabolism of other psychoactive drugs, which are also metabolized by the 2D6 enzymes resulting in their higher level. For example, inhibition of 2D6 by duloxetine may result in increased thioridazine blood concentration, which may cause cardiac arrhythmia and QTc prolongations resulting from high thioridazine plasma concentration.

Similarly, 2D6 inhibitory effects of fluoxetine and paroxetine may interfere with the biotransformation of codeine into morphine, which will result in a reduced pain relief.

The breakdown of the most important CYP enzymes is illustrated in Figure 4.1:

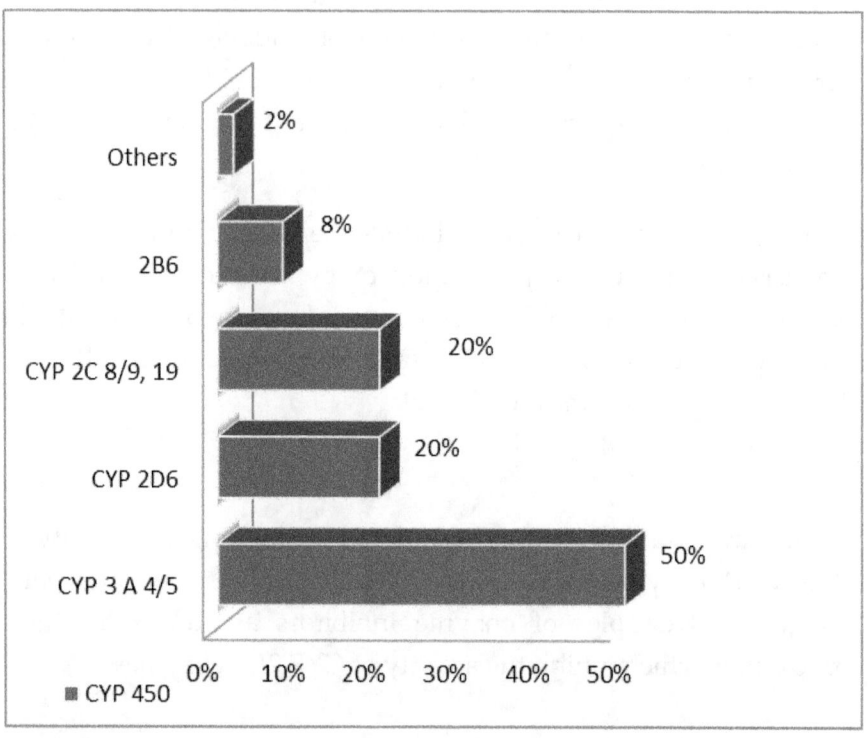

Figure 4.1: Breakdown of CYP enzyme activity. Adapted from RM Julien, CD Advokat, JE Comaty. A primer of drug action. Worth Publishers, 2011.

The production of the CYP 450 enzymes is subject to a huge genetic variation which results in a patient's clinical reaction to a psycho-active medication. For example, 7% of the white population does not have the CYP 2D6 enzymes. The result of 2D6 deficiency results in inability to metabolize drugs, which require 2D6 enzymes for their metabolism.

The lack of the 2D6 enzyme may cause hypersensitivity and higher blood levels of 2D6 metabolized drugs, and a larger side effect's profile.

Furthermore, the ingestion of two or more drugs which are metabolized by the same CYP enzyme result in competition for the CYP enzyme which may cause interference with their metabolism.

The CYP 450 3A3/4 enzyme's action can be induced by carbamazepine, which may enhance the metabolism of other psycho-active drugs metabolized by the same 3A3/4 enzymes. The enzymatic induction by carbamazepine of the CYP 3A3/4 may lower the plasma concentration of the over-the-counter medication St John's worth, and contraceptives, which are also metabolized by the CYP 3A3/4 enzymes.

Such enzymatic induction, by carbamazepine may interfere with the contraceptive efficacy and the antidepressant effect of St John's worth.

P- Glycoprotein (P-gp)

P-glycoproteins (P-gp), are glycoproteins encoded by the ABC1 gene. They are trans-membrane proteins with 6 trans- membrane domains and an additional large cytoplasmic domain containing ATP-binding sites.

The main function of P-gp is to transport a variety of substrates across the cellular membranes. They function to protect the body from harmful substances by active transportation of hydrophobic substances across the cell membrane.

The P-gp are efflux transporters located in various organ cells such as the liver, the kidneys, the adrenal glands, the placenta, the gonads, the biliary system, intestines and the brain.

P-gp activity requires energy provided by the ATP, and is capable of regulating the absorption and excretion of drugs and other substances from various body organs.

P-gp is subject to induction and inhibition similar to that of the P450 enzymes. The P-gp glycoprotein located in the gut can act as a gatekeeper and block the absorption of harmful substances and drug from the gastrointestinal system.

P-gp mechanism of action

The P-gp substrate binds to the P-gp simultaneously with one ATP molecule. The hydrolysis of the ATP shifts the substrates into a position to be excreted from the cell. The release of the phosphate from the ATP molecule occurs simultaneously with the release from the substrate. The remaining ADP then is also released from the P-gp and a new ATP molecule attaches and resets the cycle. There are more than 100 genetic variations of the P-gp glycoprotein due to a single nucleotide polymorphysm.

Woman appears to have lower hepatic P-gp levels than man, which may explain why some drugs are metabolized more efficiently by woman. The p-gp significantly affects drug pharmacokinetics by its ability to regulate the drug transport across the cell membrane. For example, increased intestinal expression of P-gp can reduce the absorption of drugs, which are P-gp substrates resulting in their lower plasma levels.

The P-gp can also facilitate the transport of compound out of the brain, across the blood brain barrier. The P-gp action is illustrated in figure 4.2:

A

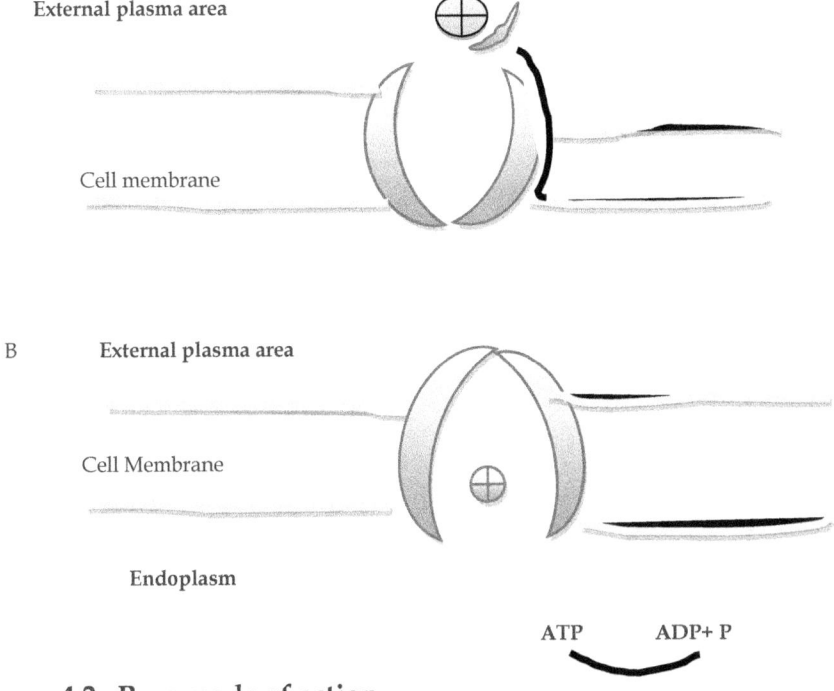

Figure 4.2: P-gp mode of action

Follows is a list of P-gp substrates, inhibitors and inducers:

P-gp substrates

Methotrexate, mitomycin, vincristine, amiodarone, atorvastatin, dilitiazem, digoxin, lovastatin, nadolol, pravastatin, propranolol, timolol, quinidine, verapamil, clarithromycin, erythromycin, fluoroquinolones,, quinine, rifampin, indinavir, ritonavir, cyclosporine, cimetidine, lidocaine, loperamide, morphine, Agomelatine, amytriptiline, citalopram, Fluoxetine, fluvoxamine, paroxetine, sertraline, venlafaxine

P-gp inhibitors

Amiodarone, diltiazem, cyclosporine, itraconazole, verapamil, verapamil, clarithromycin, erythromycin, ritonavir, cyclosporine, nifedipine, propafenone, ketoconazole, mefloquine, ofloxacin, duloxetine, citalopram, fluoxetine, fluvoxamine, imipramine, paroxetine, sertraline, trazadone, venlafaxine

P-gp inducers

Dexamethasone, phenobarbital, rifampine, St. John's wort, Antidepressants absorption and elimination from the body otgans are also influenced by the P-gp system.

Receptors

Receptors are macromolecules, which are situated in the cell membranes. Each receptor has a specific three dimensional configuration. The unique structure of each receptor determines its physical compatibility to the corresponding drug, hormone and brain neurotransmitter. Follows in figure 4.3, an illustration of the structure of a G protein-coupled receptor

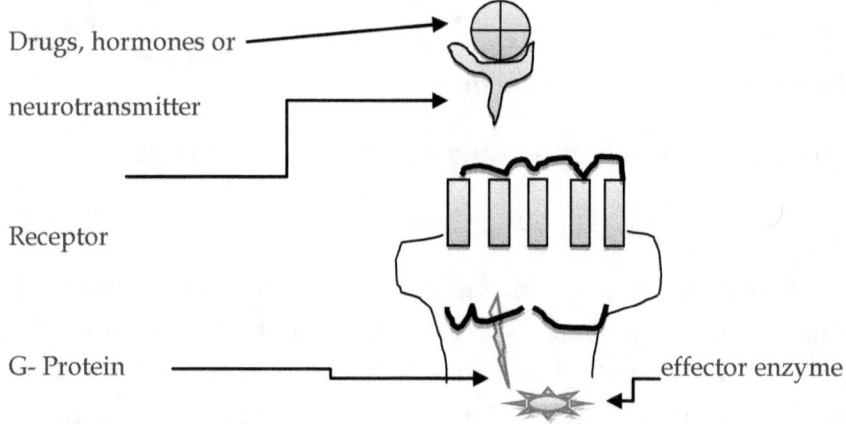

Figure 4.3: The structure of the G protein-coupled receptors.

The binding of the G protein-coupled receptor to its corresponding drug will result in an action within the cell. The receptor drug binding will activated a G protein which, in turn, will interact and will activate an effector enzyme. In the CNS there are several types of receptors. Another type of a CNS receptor is the ligand – gated ion channels. This receptor once activated is responsible for the regulation of the flow of ions across the cell membrane.

The ligand-gated receptor have a very rapid response which can last only a few milliseconds. The nicotinic receptor and the GABA receptors are examples of ligand-gated receptors which are illustrated in Figure 4.4.

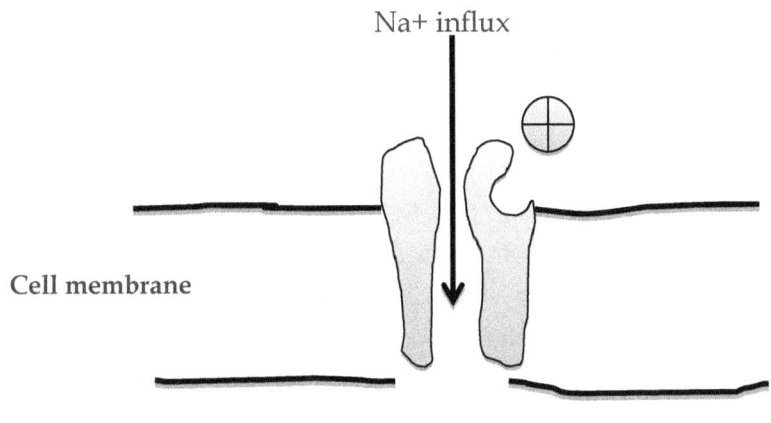

Increased intracellular Na+   (Results in cell depolarization).

Figure 4.4: Illustration of a ligand–gated receptor: The influx of the ion Na+ from the extracellular space into the endoplasm results in changes in the membrane potential and increase of the endoplasm Na+ concentration which will enhance cell depolarization. Adapted from RA Harvey, PC Champe, RD Howland, MJ Mycek. Pharmacology 3rd edition. Lippincott Williams & Wilkins, 2000.

Each receptor generates a unique response. The union between the receptor with its corresponding neurotransmitter or drug will result in either activation, inhibition or a mixed activating/ inhibition response.

Many compounds can mimic the actions of the brain neurotransmitters by binding to the same corresponding receptor which will generate a similar response to that of the original brain chemical. In general, most psycho-active drugs tend to be slightly more selective than the natural neurotransmitters.

Normally, each neurotransmitters is capable of activating only its corresponding receptors, thus creating an *agonist response*. The psycho-active drugs, on the other hand, can activate their receptors thus mimic the agonistic response of the natural neurotransmitter. Some psycho-active drugs are only **partial agonists** and activate their corresponding receptor in a lesser degree, generating a partial response. Other drugs are designed to block the receptor site and thus make the receptor unavailable to the natural neurotransmitters. Such drugs are said to have an *antagonist response*. In addition, there are designed drugs called **inverse agonist** which have an active opposite action to that of the agonist resulting in a reduced activity of the receptor below the baseline level when no agonist is present (6).

The drug actions on the nerve cell receptors can be either:

- **Agonist**: Which can generate similar effect to the natural neurotransmitter.

- **Partial agonist**: Which can generate only a partial response.

- **Antagonist**: Which can block the effects of the natural neurotransmitter.

- **Inverse agonist**: Which can generate an opposite effect to that of the agonist drug.

External signals can activate the cell DNA to produce the cell membrane receptors by the activating the corresponding gene.

Receptors can be removed from the surface of the cell membrane, back into the cell and destroyed by lysosomes to make space for newly-formed receptors.

The number of the cell receptor can be either up regulated or down regulated by external modulators. Nurotransmitters, for instance, can regulate their own receptor's quantity either by activating or inhibiting the DNA.

The continuous administration of an agonist or antagonist may lead to changes in the receptor's responsiveness, making the receptor desensitized to the drug action. Voltage gated receptors require rest period (latency) following stimulation before they can be activated again. During the recovery period, the voltage gated receptors are refractory or unresponsive (5).

An important method to evaluate receptor activity is the dose-response curve, which describes the amount of biological responses for a given drug dose (1). At a low dose, the drug effect is low due to the low number of occupied receptors. On the other hand, at a higher dose, a bigger number of receptors are occupied resulting in a greater biological response.

Psychopharmacology references

1 Meyer JS, Quenzer LF: Psychopharmacology: Drugs, the brain and behaviour. Sinauer Association, Inc., 2005.

2 Julien RM, Advokat CD, Comaty JE. A primer of drug action. Worth Publishers, 2011.

3 Rang HP, Dale MM, Ritter JM, Moore PK. Pharmacology, fifth

edition Churchill Livingstone, 2003.

4 Nestler EJ, Hyman SE, Malenka RC. Molecular Nwuropharmacology. A foundation for clinical neuroscience. 2nd edition.McGraw Hill, 2009.

5 Harvey RA, Champe PC, Howland RD, Mycek MJ. Pharmacology 3rd edition. Lippincott Williams & Wilkins, 2000.

6 Stahl's Essential Psychopharmacology. Third edition. Cambridge University Press, 2008.

5

Agomelatine

Brand name: Valdoxane

Mode of action: agomelatine

1. Agomelatine is a potent melatonin MT1 and melatonin MT2 receptors <u>agonist</u>:

The majority of the MT1 receptors are located in the pituitary gland, and in the suprachiasmatic area of the hypothalamus. Activation of the MT1 receptors facilitates sleep, while the activation of the MT2 receptors, which are predominantly located in the retina, facilitate the phase shift circadian rhythms.

The activation of both MT1 and MT2 receptors result in re synchronization of the circadian rhythms, while the inhibition of the melatonin MT1 and MT2 receptors result in de-synchronization of the body's circadian rhythms.

Circadian rhythms are physical and mental changes that have a 24-hour cycle and are controlled by a master clock that consists of a group of nerve cells which are situated in the suprachiasmatic nucleus (SCN) located in the hypothalamus.

The presence or absence of light is the principal cue which influences and regulates the circadian rhythms.

The human circadian rhythms consist of the sleep – wake cycle, cortisol secretion, glucose homeostasis, metabolism and body temperature.

The circadian rhythms are controlled by two genes located in the suprachiasmatic nucleus (SCN): **BMAL1** and **Clock**. When both genes become active, they activate the expression of two intracellular proteins: **Per** and **Cry** which dimerize and then exit the nucleus and move into the cytoplasm. In the cell cytoplasm, the dimerized Per and Cry become phosphorylated and inhibit the BMAL1 and clock genes' expression via a negative feedback loop.

Once the phosphorylated Per and Cry proteins are degraded by a kinase the transcription of BMAL1 and Clock will start all over again.

Light stimuli transmitted to the SCN via the retinohypotalamic tract affects the expression of the circadian rhythm central pacemaker. The SCN has high concentration of melatonin MT1 and MT2 as well as 5-HT2C receptors. The binding of melatonin to the MT1 and MT2 receptors in the SCN, suppresses neuronal firing and facilitates sleep.

Melatonin supplement is used to facilitate the readjustment of the light – dark shifts that occurr in jet lag and shift work (2).

Abnormal circadian rhythm is associated with sleep disorders, depression and seasonal affective disorder.

2. Agomelatine is a 5–HT2C <u>antagonist:</u>

The 5-HT2C receptors are located in the frontal cortex, hippocampus and in the basal ganglia. The 5-HT2C receptors have a tonic inhibitory effect on dopamine and norepinephrine in the frontal cortex. The inhibition of the 5-HT2C receptors has been shown to increase extracellular levels of dopamine and norepinephrine in the frontal cortex (3).

In addition, agomelatine affects the following receptors:

- ✓ **Anticholinergic(Ach) muscarinic receptors affinity: No effect**: Agomelatine has negligible side effects of dry mouth, constipation, blurred vision and drowsiness.

- ✓ **Histaminergic (H1) receptors affinity: No effect.** Agomelatine has negligible side effects of sedation and weight gain.

- ✓ **Adrenergic (α 1) receptors affinity: No effect.** Agomelatine has negligible side effects of hypotension, dizziness, drowsiness and other cardiovascular effects.

Pharmacokinetics of agomelatine

Agomelatine has **linear pharmacokinetics.** Thus any dose change of agomelatine leads to a proportional change in agomelatine plasma levels. Food intake does not modify the absorption rates and the bioavailability of agomelatine.

Peak plasma levels (Tmax): 1 - 2 hours.

As side effects of any drug are dose-related and tend to emerge at the peak of its plasma levels, a single dose of agomelatine may result in emerging side effects within 1 hours of agomelatine ingestion.

It appears that female and elderly patients show higher plasma levels.

Steady state: Agomelatine reaches a plasma steady state concentration within **5 – 7 days** of daily regular use.

Absorption: >80%. Agomelatine is well absorbed (>80%) by the gastrointestinal tract. It appears that the presence of food may minimally slow agomelatine absorption.

Protein binding: 95%. Agomelatine is highly a protein bound. More than 95% of the plasma circulating agomelatine is attached to plasma protein: 35% to albumin and 35% to acid glycoprotein.

Bioavailability: <5%

Agomelatine bioavailability is very low <5% at the therapeutic oral dose.

Half-life (t 1/2): 2-3 Hours

Volume of distribution: 35 L

Metabolism: Agomelatine is primarily metabolised by the liver via three CYP 450 enzymes: The CYP **1A2, 2C9 and 2C19**

Agomelatine has two principal **inactive metabolites**: *The 7-o-demethylated agomelatine* and the *hydroxylate agomelatine*. Both metabolites are rapidly conjugated and eliminated in the urine.

The P-gp System

Agomelatine is a **P-gp substrate** and may have the potential to increase the bioavailability of co- administered compounds that are also substrates of the P-gp transport system.

Elimination: Urine 80%, Faeces 20%

Agomelatine clearance is drastically reduced in patients with liver and renal impairment. Liver impairment patients may experience 100 times increase in agomelatine plasma levels, while patients with renal impairment may experience up to 25% increase in agomelatine plasma levels.

How supplied

Agomelatine supplied in Tablets of 25mg

Dose range

For depression: 25 – 50 mg once daily at bedtime.

Agomelatine clinical indications

- Major depression
- Generalised anxiety disorder
- Sleep disturbances

Major Depressive Disorder (MDD)

The efficacy of agomelatine for the treatment of major depression showed comparable efficacy to that of other antidepressants and greater than placebo.

In addition, agomelatine has better remission rates compared to placebo (6) as illustrated in Figure 5.1

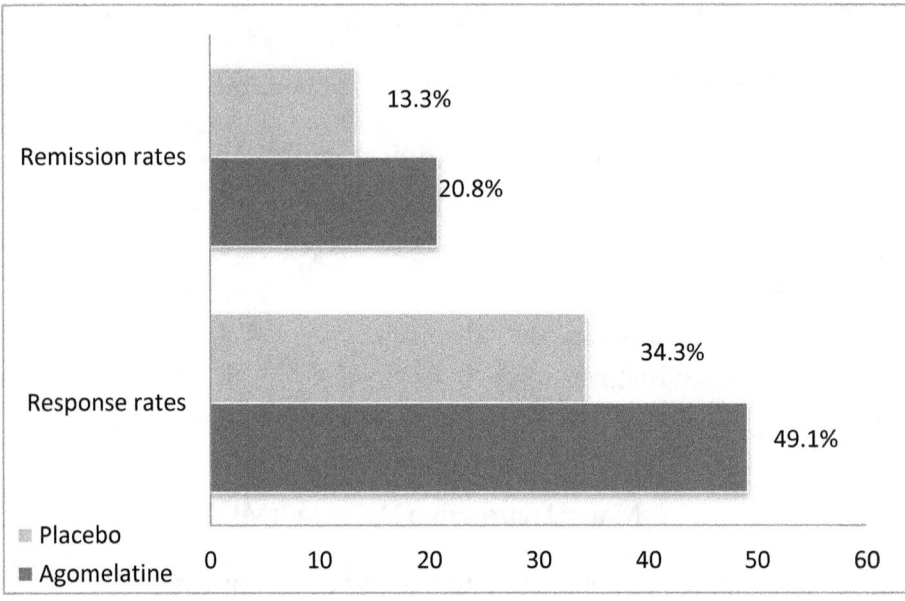

Figure 5.1: Agomelatine response and remission rates compared to placebo. Response defined as >50% improvement from baseline Hamilton Rating scale for depression (HAM-D) and Remission defined as HAM-D score of <6 after 8 weeks of treatment with agomelatine 25mg/day or with placebo. Data adapted from Kennedy SH, Emsley R. Randomized, double-blind, placebo controlled trial of agomelatinein in the treatment of MDD. Dose ranging trial versus placebo. Eur. Neuropsychopharmacology. 2006:16:93-100.

How to treat with agomelatine

For the treatment of major Depression (MDD): Start with 25mg of agomelatine at bedtime. The dose can be increased, up to a maximum of 50mg after 2 weeks of treatment.

When and how to take medication

Agomelatine should be taken at bedtime as a once-a-day dose. Do not break or chew the medication as it might interfere with the drug pharmacokinetics.

How to stop agomelatine

A sudden discontinuation of agomelatine was not associated with discontinuation syndrome. However, a slow tapering of the drug is still recommended.

How long it takes to get an antidepressant effect

In order to get an antidepressant effect, agomelatine should be used daily for at least 2 – 4 weeks. Like all the other antidepressants, agomelatine needs time before a substantial mood improvement emerges.

Side effects of agomelatine

Most side effects of agomelatine develop at the beginning of the treatment and commonly subside with time. The most troubling side effects of agomelatine are **headache**, and **nightmares.**

Nervous system: Activation is a common side effects which is associated with agomelatine use. Other CNS side effects include:

- somnolence
- sedation
- Fatigue
- headache
- Insomnia
- agitation
- anxiety
- vivid dreams
- dizziness

- *seizures* (very rare)
- rash

Gastro intestinal: (GI) side effects are less common with agomelatine use. The most common GI side effects of agomelatine include:

- decreased appetite
- nausea ,
- vomiting
- dry mouth
- diarrhea
- constipation
- upper abdominal pain

Sexual : Agomelatine is associated with lower incidence of **sexual dysfunction** . The most common sexual related side effects of agomelatine include:

- decreased sex drive
- delayed ejaculation
- Impotence
- abnormal orgasm

Agomelatine side effect that need immediate attention

- Confusion
- Excitation
- Onset of seizure
- Yellow skin / eyes
- Fatigue
- Severe allergic reaction
- Irregular heart beats
- Hypertension

- Hypotension
- Induction of manic or hypomanic episode
- Activation of suicidal ideation and behaviour

Physical & psychological dependence

Patients using agomelatine did not show any tendencies for drug seeking behaviour. However, patients with a history of drug abuse should be closely monitored for signs of agomelatine misuse or abuse, which includes drug seeking behavior, development of tolerance and requests for dose increase.

Agomelatine discontinuation reaction

A sudden discontinuation of agomelatine is not associated with a discontinuation reaction.

Safety profile of agomelatine

Use in pregnancy: Safety Unknown

Reproductive studies with agomelatine in rats and rabbit showed no effect on fertility, embryo foetal development and pre-and post- natal development. In addition, genotoxicity assays showed no mutagenic or clastogenic potential with agomelatine.

However, the effect of agomelatine on human embryos is unknown.

The risk of pregnant mothers with a history of depression to develop depression during their pregnancy and especially after child delivery is very high and often requires the continuation of the treatment with SSRIs during and after the pregnancy.

Equally important, the use of agomelatine in the last trimester of pregnancy may be associated with a higher incidence of respiratory distress and pulmonary hypertension, cyanosis, apnea, seizures, temperature instability, vomiting, hypoglycemia, hypotonia, hyperreflexia, tremor, irritability, constant crying and jitteriness, which may require prolonged hospitalization, tube feeding and respiratory support.

There is increased risk for the newborn to develop Persistent Newborn Pulmonary Hypertension (PPHN), when agomelatine is used during the last trimester of pregnancy, and it is associated with substantial neonatal morbidity and mortality. The risk of developing PPHN was six-fold higher in infants exposed to SSRI after the 20th week of gestation.

Thus, the use of agomelatine during the first trimester as well as throughout the pregnancy is not recommended.

Use during lactation

Agomelatine secretion in the human breast milk is unknown. Agomelatine and its metabolites are excreted in the milk of lactating rats.

As all psychotropic medications are known to be secreted in the breast milk, it is recommended to discontinue with breast feeding due to unknown effects of agomelaine on the newborn's normal growth and development.

Carcinogenesis

In carcinogenicity studies, agomelatine induced an increase in the incidence of liver tumors in rats and mouse at doses 110- fold higher than that of the therapeutic dose. In addition, there was an increase in the frequency of benign mammary fibro- adenomas in rats exposed to agomelatine at does 60-fold higher than the therapeutic dose.

Avoid using agomelatine in the following cases:

- In patients taking MAOI medication.

- Proven allergy to agomelatine.
- History of seizure.

Drug interaction

Drug interaction may develop as the result of agomelatine metabolism by the liver enzymes CYP 450: **1A2, 2C9, 2C19**. Table 4.1 shows agomelatine drug interactions.

Follow a list of agomelatine drug interactions.

- **Fluvoxamine:** The concomitant use of agomelatine with fluvoxamine increases agomelatine plasma levels by **44 – fold** due to its inhibition of its metabolism.
- **Omeprazol:** The concomitant use of agomelatine with omeprazole (a 1A2 inducer) can **decrease** agomelatine blood levels.
- **Nicotine:** The concomitant use of agomelatine with nicotine (a 1A2 inducer) can **decrease** agomelatine blood levels.
- **MAOI:** The concomitant use of agomelatine with MAOI can lead to CNS toxicity and serotonin syndrome. Wait 21 days after MAOI was stopped before initiating treatment with agomelatine. Wait 5-7 days to start MAOI after discontinuing agomelatine.
- **Tramadol:** The concomitant use of agomelatine with tramadol may increase the risk to develop seizures.
- **Oestrogen:** The concomitant use of agomelatine with oestrogen can increase agomelatine blood levels.
- **Paroxetine:** The concomitant use of agomelatine with paroxetine may increase agomelatine blood levels.

Warnings for agomelatine

> **Pregnancy: Risk category unknown.** Try to avoid the use of agomelatine during pregnancy or breastfeeding.

Assessment of the risk versus benefits must be discussed with the patient.

- **Agomelatine may cause an increase in suicidal risk in young adults.** Pooled analysis of trials of drugs used for MDD showed that SNRIs and SSRIs may increase the risk of suicidal thinking and behavior in children, adolescents and young adults aged 18-24. The use of antidepressants in this population must balance the risk of suicide with the clinical need. Careful monitoring of the patient's clinical worsening, and suicidality should also involve the family and all other caregivers for the increase in suicidal risk in this population.
- **Serotonin syndrome** may develop with agomelatine use. Serotonin syndrome symptoms may include agitation, dizziness, hallucinations, delirium, seizures and coma along with autonomic instability that includes tachycardia, fluctuating blood pressure, flushing, hyperthermia, tremor, muscular rigidity, myoclonus, hyperreflexia, incoordination. The concomitant use of agomelatine with MAOI may precipitate serotonin syndrome which may be fatal.
- **Activation of hypomania or mania:** May occurred in agomelatine-treated bipolar patients. As agomelatine may trigger mania in predisposed patients, it should be used with caution in patients with a history of bipolar mood disorder.
- **Seizure:** The risk of seizure is relatively low with agomelatine. However, the co-administration of agomelatine with tramadol may increase seizure risk.
- **Alcohol abuse:** Agomelatine is not recommended in patient abusing alcohol.
- **Liver impairment**: Agomelatine should be avoided in people with liver cirrhosis and liver insufficiency.

Agomelatine dose should be reduced in patients with liver impairment.

- ➢ **Hepato-biliary disorder**: Agomelatine may increase the liver enzymes ALAT > 3 times the upper limit of the normal range. It may increase the liver enzyme GGT >3 times the upper limit of the normal range. Increased alkaline phosphatase >3 times the upper limit of the normal rang was also observed with agomelatine use.
- ➢ **Liver injury risk factors**: Caution should be exercised when prescribing agomelatine in patients with risk factors of liver injury such as alcoholism, diabetes, and obesity.
- ➢ **Monitoring liver function**: Cases of liver failure, elevation of liver enzymes exceeding 10 times the normal upper limits, hepatitis and jaundice have been reported with agomelatine use. Most cases occurred during the first month of treatment with agomelatine. The increase in serum transaminase usually returned to normal levels upon drug discontinuation. **Liver function test should be performed in all patient at the initiation of treatment with agomelatine and then periodically after 3 weeks, 6 weeks, 12 weeks, and in 24 weeks.** Any dose increase of agomelatine requires new liver function test to be performed at the same frequency as when initiating treatment. **Any increase in serum transaminase requires urgent liver function test which must be repeated within 48hours.** Treatment with agomelatine must be discontinued if the serum transaminase exceeds 3X the upper normal limit. Patient developing symptoms of liver injury such as dark urine, light coloured stool, yellow skin, yellow eyes, pain in the upper right belly and onset of severe fatigue require immediate treatment discontinuation and urgent liver transaminase monitoring.

- ➢ **Kidney impairment**: Agomelatine should be used with caution in patients with renal impairment and require a lower dose.
- ➢ **MAOI:** Agomelatine combined with MAOI may be fatal. Agomelatine requires **7 day** washout period before starting with MAOI. Agomelatine requires **3 week** washout period after MAOI was stopped.

Agomelatine overdose

General symptoms of agomelatine overdose

Initially, the patient may feel extremely tired and lethargic. The pulse will slow down, and the breathing frequency will also reduce.

As the level of intoxication increases, the level of consciousness will decrease, and the patient will become unresponsive to external stimulations.

The reflexes will disappear, and breathing will get shallower. The patient's pulse and blood pressure will decrease until the cardiovascular system collapse.

Agomelatine is **relatively safe in monotherapy overdose;** it is associated with low incidence of fatalities. Overdosed patient with 2450mg of agomelatine had a full spontaneous recovery without any cardiovascular-related problems. However, the concomitant use of agomelatine with alcohol and with other central nervous depressants such as painkillers or benzo- diazepines may result in a death cause by respiratory depression.

Specific symptoms of agomelatine over dose are

- over sedation
- somnolence
- agitation

- anxiety
- tension
- dizziness
- fatigue
- disorientation
- seizure
- vomiting
- cyanosis
- loss of consciousness

What to do in the case of overdose

In general, there is no antidote for agomelatine overdose and the management is mainly supportive, aimed to maintaining respiration, pulse and blood pressure.

In the event of a recent overdose with agomelatine a stomach washout might help to eliminate the un- absorbed drug from the stomach. Stomach washout is conducted with a large – bore orogastric tube and also requires appropriate airway protection. The aim of the stomach lavage is to get rid of the drug leftovers.

In many ER departments, active charcoal is used to treat poisonings and overdose following oral ingestion of agomelatine.

The active charcoal has a high degree of micro porosity and huge surface area, which reversibly binds to the ingested toxin and alcohol and prevents their absorption from the gastrointestinal tract.

Active charcoal comes in a plastic tube of 25 grams premixed with water and is given only once.

Administration of activated charcoal can decrease the Cmax and

AUC by an average of one-third.

In some ER departments, ipecac is also used in order to induce vomiting of the ingested toxin, however **induction of emesis is not recommended in comatose patients**.

Due to the large volume of distribution of agomelatine, forced diuresis, dialysis hemoperfusion and exchange transfusion are unlikely to be effective. Keeping the patient's airway patent is compulsory, especially in semi-comatose individuals. The patient should be placed on his side in order to prevent aspiration of the vomitus. Suffocation due to vomit is the leading cause of death in agomelatine overdose. Blood pressure and heart rate monitoring is very important. Fluid intake should be monitored with intravenous infusion of saline. Urinary output should be also carefully monitored. In most cases, agomelatine overdose, requires hospitalization of the patient for at least 24 hours for intense observation.

Agomelatine references

1 Stahl SM. Valdoxan: A novel antidepressant. Arbor Scientia 2011.

2 Arendt J, Skene DJ, Middleton B eta al. Efficacy of melatonin treatment in jet lag, shift work and blindness. J Biol Rhythms. 1997:12:604-617.

3 Stahl SM. Essential Psychopharmacology of depression and bipolar disorders. Cambridge University Press. 2000.

4 Akamine, Yumiko,Yasui-Furukori et al. Psychotropic drug – drug interactions involving P-gp. Nov 2012 Vol 26 issue 11- 959 – 973.

5 Weiss j, Dormann SM, Martin- Facklam et al. Inhibition of P-gp by newer antidepressants. J. Pharmacol Exp Ther. Apr 2003; 305(1):197-204.

6 Kennedy SH, Emsley R. Placebo controlled trial of agomelatine in the treatment of MDD. Eur. Neuropsychopharmacology. 2006:16:93-100.

6

Bupropion

Brand name: Wellbutrin

Mode of action of bupropion:

1. Bupropion is a Norepinephrine reuptake transporter (NET) antagonist: The inhibition of the norepinephrine reuptake transporter (NET), located on the presynaptic neurons, by bupropion, results in increased norepinephrine levels. The inhibition of NET by bupropion is 65-fold less potent than that of imipramine.

2. Bupropion is a dopamine reuptake transporter (DAT) antagonist: The inhibition of the dopamine reuptake transporter (DAT), located on the presynaptic neurons, by bupropion, results in increased dopamine in the frontal cortex. It appears that bupropion is twice as potent a DAT antagonist than a (NET) antagonist. Bupropion DAT inhibition is 100% compared to NET inhibition being between 22% - 35%.

3. Bupropion is a nicotinic acetylcholine receptors α3β4 antagonist: The α3β4 is a nicotinic Ach receptor which is located in the CNS as well as at the neuromuscular junctions, autonomic ganglia and at the adrenal medulla. This group of receptors are ligand-gated ion channels. Their activation by acetyl choline leads to a rapid influx of Na^+ and Ca^+ into the cell endoplasm, which leads to a cellular depolarization. The depolarization effect is rapidly desensitized. The nicotinic receptors are made of five subunits organized around a central pore. To date, 11 heterologous subunits of the α3β4 have been identified. Eight are α subunits and three are β subunits. The α3β4 receptor plays an important role in arousal, cognition, attention and memory (1). In addition, the nicotinic receptor has a strong affinity for nicotine, a highly addictive substance. The ability of bupropion to block the α3β4 nicotinic receptors may be relevant to the bupropion's role in nicotine addiction.

The selective effects of bupropion on the anticholinergic, histaminergic and α adrenergic receptors are summarized as follows:

- ✓ **Anticholinergic Ach muscarinic affinity: Low.** Bupropion has low side effects of dry mouth, constipation, blurred vision and drowsiness.

- ✓ **Histaminergic H1 affinity: Low.** Bupropion has low side effects of sedation and weight gain.

- ✓ **adrenergic α1 affinity: Low.** Bupropion has low side effects of hypotension, dizziness, drowsiness and other cardiovascular effects.

Pharmacokinetics of Bupropion

Bupropion has **linear pharmacokinetics,** and it appears to induce its own metabolism. Any dose increase of bupropion may lead to a proportionate increase in its plasma levels. Thus, the higher the daily dose of bupropion, the higher the plasma level will get.

Peak plasma levels (Tmax):

- (IR) Immediate release formulation: **2 hours**
- XL formulation: **5 hours**.
- Bupropion metabolite: up to **43 hours**

Steady State: Steady-state plasma level will develop within 8 days. Steady-state is often associated with a significant reduction of side effect's symptoms. Adolescent females have been shown to have higher bupropion plasma concentration and longer bupropion half-life, which might explain the higher risk of seizure in young adolescent females.

Absorption: Bupropion is well absorbed by the gastrointestinal system and *it is not affected by the presence of food.*

Half-Life (T ½): 12-14 hours

Protein binding: 80% 80% of the bupropion is bound to albumin. Although the parent compound has a relatively short half-life, bupropion active metabolite has a much longer half-life, which reduces the risk of discontinuation syndrome.

Bioavailability: 20% in animals no studies conducted in humans.

Metabolism: CYP 450: 2D6, 2B6

Bupropion is primarily metabolized in the liver by the CYP 450 enzymes. Bupropion is a **2B6 substrates and a strong 2D6 inhibitor.** Bupropion is metabolized into three major metabolites: *Hydroxybupropion, Threohyrobupropion and Erythrohydrobupropion.* Out of the three metabolites, the S-S hydroxybupropion has been shown to possess significant biological activity. Bupropion's active metabolites can accumulate in the plasma to levels that are higher than that of the parent compound.

Bupropion's metabolism displays high variability. It appears that the metabolism of bupropion can vary up to 7-fold, in the same person, which can increase bupropion's half-life from 12 to 38 hours. Furthermore, patients treated with agents that are also metabolized by the liver enzyme 2D6 require a lower dose of the concomitant medication.

In addition, patients with liver disease can experience a significant decrease in bupropion metabolism, which might lead to bupropion accumulation in the blood.

The P-gp System

Bupropion effects on the P-gp system is **unknown.** However it may have the potential to increase bioavailability of co-administered compounds that are substrate of the P-gp system.

Elimination: Urine 80%, 20% Faeces.

How supplied

- Bupropion IR Tablets: 75mg, 100mg.
- Bupropion XL: 150mg, 300mg
- Buproprion SR: 100mg, 150mg, 200mg

Dose range

- Bupropion XL: For depression 150mg – 450mg once daily.
- Bupropion SR: 200mg – 450mg in 2 divided doses.
- Bupropion IR: 150-450mg/day

Bupropion clinical indications

- Major depression
- Nicotine addiction
- ADHD?

Major Depressive Disorder (MDD)

Bupropion showed comparable efficacy to that of other antidepressants in the treatment of major depression. Several studies have found that bupropion response rates was 60% compared to 30% of placebo (4).

In addition, combination of bupropion with SSRI gained substantial popularity as an effective augmentation of its antidepressant effects.

Furthermore, bupropion showed reduced propensity to induce mania in bipolar patients. However, like all antidepressants, bupropion use in bipolar patients should be monitored for the risk of inducing mania or hypomania.

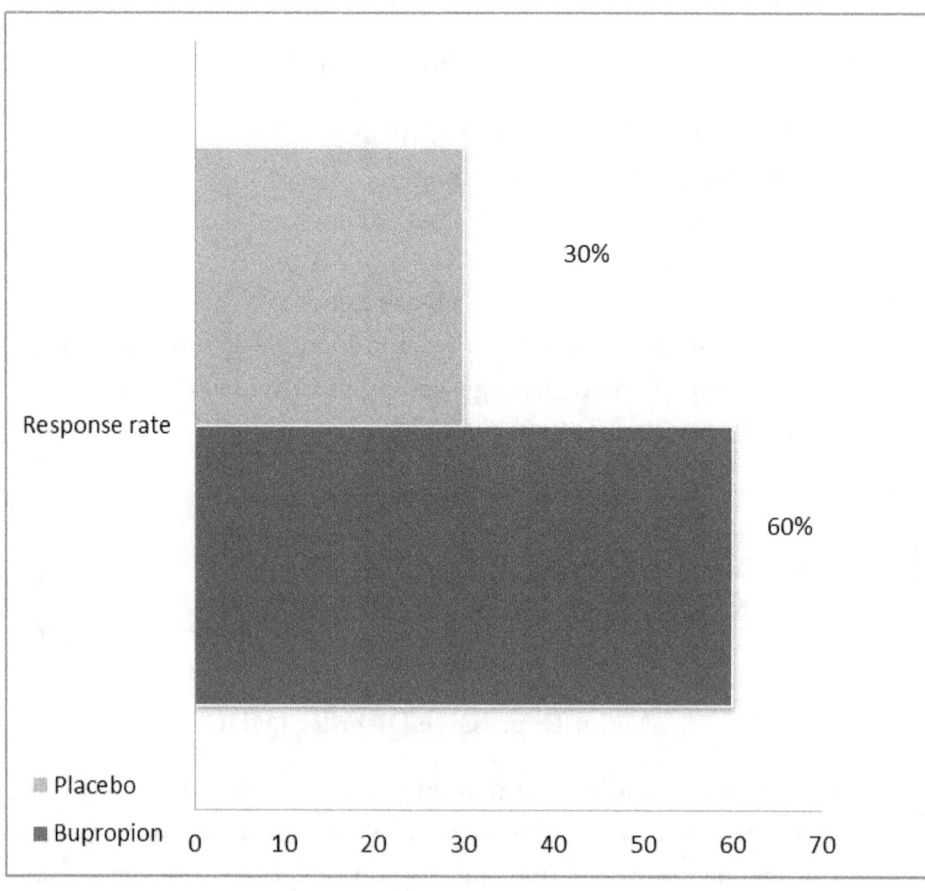

Figure 6.1: Bupropion response rate compared to placebo. Response defined as >50% improvement from the baseline Hamilton Rating scale for depression (HAM-D).

Adapted from: Zung WWK, Brodie HKH, Fabre L et al.: Comparative efficacy and safety of bupropion and placebo in the treatment of depression. Psychopharmacology (Berl) 1983, 79:343-347.

Smoking cessation

Bupropion was shown to be effective in helping people stop smoking and in reducing cigarette consumption.

Special indications

- ➢ **Attention deficit Disorder ADHD** Bupropion was shown to be effective and well- tolerated in children and adolescent with ADHD. Currently the use of bupropion should be reserved as second-line agent for children with ADHD.
- ➢ **Obesity:** Bupropion SR showed some promising results in weight reduction when compared to placebo.
- ➢ **Fatigue:** Bupropion showed some promising results in the treatment of fatigue.

How to treat with bupropion

For treatment of Major Depression (MDD)

- **XL formula**: Start with bupropion XL 150mg once a day in the morning to be increase to 300mg once a day after 4 days. In severe cases, a maximum of 450mg can be given once daily.
- **SR formula**: Start with bupropion SR initial dose of 100mg twice a day to be increased after 3 days up to 150mg twice a day to a maximum of 400mg a day only in severe unresponsive cases.

- **For nicotine addiction:** Start with bupropion SR 150mg once a day to be increased after 3 days to 150mg twice a day, usually for a period of 7-12 weeks. The maximum dose should not exceed 300mg a day. Start with treatment at least 1 week before cessation of smoking.

When and how to take medication

Preferably take bupropion in the morning for the once-a-day dose for the XL formulation. Doses above 450mg carry a higher risk for seizure. Do not break or chew the SR or the XL medication as it might interfere with the drug pharmacokinetics.

How to stop bupropion

Although there are no reports of withdrawal symptoms following bupropion cessation, a slow tapering of bupropion is recommended. In the event of getting withdrawal symptoms reinstate the previous bupropion dose, and once the symptoms disappear, start reducing the bupropion dose at a slower taper and over longer period of time.

How long it takes to get an antidepressant effect

In order to get an antidepressant effect, bupropion should be used for at least 2 – 4 weeks. Although studies did not show increased efficacy above 300 mg a day, some patients might benefit from the higher dose of 450 mg a day.

Side effects of bupropion

Most of bupropion's side effects are probably related to its ability to increase norepinephrine and dopamine in the brain.

They are dose related and often develop soon after the initiation of treatment and subside with time. The most common side effects of bupropion are:

Nervous system

- Agitation
- Insomnia
- Restlessness
- Muscle pain
- Tremor
- Hot flushes
- Headache
- Dizziness
- *Seizures* (more common in predisposed individuals and with immediate release formulation)
- Increased sweating
- Fatigue
- Somnolence
- Rash
- Blurred vision

Gastro intestinal System: Bupropion's GI side effects are highly common and can develop within 30 minutes of bupropion ingestion. They are more likely the result of the direct effect of bupropion on the intestinal mucosa than of its peak plasma level.

- *Decreased appetite*
- Weight loss
- Nausea
- Vomiting
- Dry mouth
- Diarrhea
- Constipation
- *Possible weight loss*
- Gastritis

Sexual Bupropion use is associated with lower incidence of sexual dysfunction. Bupropion's most common sexual side effects are

- Decreased sex drive
- Delayed ejaculation
- Impotence
- Abnormal orgasm

Buproprion side effects that need immediate attention

- Confusion
- Excitation
- Onset of seizure
- Yellow skin / eyes
- Severe allergic reaction
- Irregular heart beats
- Hypertension
- Induction of manic or hypomanic episode
- Activation of suicidal ideation and behaviour

Physical & psychological dependence

Bupropion users showed some increase in motor activity, agitation and excitement. In addition, patients with a history of drug abuse, the use of bupropion was associated with mild amphetamine-like activity with increased feeling of euphoria and drug desirability.

Animal studies with bupropion have shown some similarity to psychostimulants, which included increased motor activity, mild stereotyped behavioral response as well as increased rates of responding in several schedules-controlled behaviour paradigms.

Therefore, patients with a history of drug abuse should be closely monitored for signs of bupropion misuse or abuse, which include drug seeking behavior, development of tolerance and requests for dose increase.

Bupropion discontinuation reaction

A sudden discontinuation of bupropion may be associated with a discontinuation reaction which is self-limiting. The most common symptoms of bupropion discontinuation reaction are:

- Irritability
- Agitation
- Dizziness
- Electric shock sensations
- Anxiety
- Confusion
- Headache
- Lethargy
- Insomnia
- Seizures
- Dysphoric mood

A slow down-titration of bupropion is often reduce the risk of having the discontinuation reaction

Safety profile of bupropion

Use in pregnancy: FDA risk category C

According the FDA the risk for using bupropion during pregnancy is **risk category is C** (i.e.: some animal studies showed adverse effects but there are no controlled studies in humans). The risk of pregnant mothers with a history of depression to develop depression during their pregnancy and especially after child delivery is very high and often requires the continuation of the treatment with SSRIs during and after the pregnancy.

Studies performed in rabbits at doses 11 times the maximum human dose (MRHD), resulted in a slightly increased incidence of fetal malformation and skeletal variations, as well as decreased fetal weight. In a human pregnancy study with bupropion, 1200 infants with bupropion exposure during pregnancy showed no greater risk for congenital malformation or cardiovascular malformation following exposure to bupropion in the first trimester. The use of bupropion in the last trimester of pregnancy is associated, (as with all other antidepressants), with higher incidence of respiratory distress and pulmonary hypertension, cyanosis, apnea, seizures, temperature instability vomiting, hypoglycemia, hypotonia, hyperreflexia, tremor, irritability, constant crying and jitteriness, which required prolonged hospitalization, tube feeding and respiratory support.

There is an increased possibility of PPHN in the newborn, which is associated with substantial neonatal morbidity and mortality. The risk of developing PPHN was six-fold higher in infants exposed to SSRI after the 20th week of gestation. It appears that the risk of getting PPHN is common to all SSRIs used during the pregnancy.

Thus, the use of bupropion during the first trimester as well as throughout the pregnancy is not recommended.

Use during lactation

Bupropion is secreted in the breast milk. Due to its unknown effects on the newborn's normal growth and development, breast feeding should be avoided.

Carcinogenesis

There is no evidence of carcinogenesis with the use of bupropion in treated rats with a daily dose up to 7 times the maximum recommended human dose (MRHD).

In addition, no liver lesions nor liver tumors were observed in mouse studies.

Avoid using bupropion in the following cases

- Recent head injury
- History of seizure
- Current or past history of anorexia
- Current or past history of bulimia
- Alcohol withdrawal
- Brain tumor
- Proven allergy to bupropion

Follow a drug interaction list of bupropion. The drug interaction is related to its metabolism by the liver enzymes CYP 450: 2D6 and 1A2

- **L-Dopa:** concomitant use increased excitement, restlessness, nausea and tremor due to the increased dopamine in the brain.
- **Imipramine & nortriptyline:** Concomitant use Increased imipramine blood levels by 57%, and increased nortriptyline blood levels by 200% which may be associated with increased risk for seizures.
- **Fluoxetine; Concomitant use:** May cause delirium, panic and myoclonus.
- **Venlafaxine:** Concomitant use may cause 3-fold increase in the venlafaxine levels.
- **MAOI :** Concomitant use may cause CNS toxicity- serotonin syndrome. Wait 21 days after MAOI was stopped before initiating treatment with bupropion. In

addition wait 5-7 days to start MAOI after discontinuing bupropion.
- **Tramadol & Codeine:** Concomitant use may Increased seizures and interfere with the analgesic action of codeine.
- **Quinolone:** Concomitant use may cause seizures.
- **Zolpidem:** concomitant use May cause visual hallucinations.
- **Pseudoepohedrine:** Concomitant use May cause seizures and manic-like reactions.
- **Metropolol:** Concomitant use may Increased metropolol plasma levels.
- **Thioridazine:** Concomitant use may cause cardiac arrhythmias due to 2D6 inhibition by buproprion.

Warning & Precautions

> **Pregnancy**: **Risk category C**. Try to avoid bupropion use during pregnancy or breastfeeding. Assessment of the risk versus benefits must be discussed with the patient.

> **Bupropion may cause an increase in suicidal risk in young adults**. Pooled analysis of trials of drugs used for MDD showed that SNRIs and SSRIs may increase the risk of suicidal thinking and behavior in children, adolescents and young adults aged 18-24. The use of antidepressants in this population must balance the risk of suicide with the clinical need. Careful monitoring of the patient's clinical worsening, and suicidality should also involve the family and all other caregivers.

> **Suicide:** The FDA requires all antidepressants to carry a black box warning stating that antidepressant may increase the risk for suicide in persons under the age of 25 years. This warning is based on data suggesting that suicide ideations and behavior has a 2-fold increase in

children and in adolescents, and 1.5-fold increase in the 18 – 24 age group.
- **Serotonin syndrome** may develop with bupropion use. Serotonin syndrome symptoms may include agitation, dizziness, hallucinations, delirium, seizures and coma along with autonomic instability which include tachycarfia, fluctuating blood pressure, flushing, hyperthermia, tremor, muscular rigidity, myoclonus, hyperreflexia, incoordination. The concomitant use of bupropion with MAOI may precipitate serotonin syndrome which may be fatal.
- **Activation of hypomania or mania** may occurr in bupropion-treated bipolar patients. As bupropion may trigger mania in the predisposed patients, it should be used cautiously in patients with a history of bipolar mood disorder.
- **Seizure**: bupropion is associated with a dose-related risk of seizures. Bupropion immediate release carries a risk of seizure of 0.4% at doses below 450mg/day (which is 2-4 times higher than that of an SSRI). The risk of seizure is increased in patients with a history of seizure and head trauma as well as with the concomitant use of medications which lower seizure threshold, such as tramadol, alcohol, opiates, cocaine, over the counter stimulants, anorectics, systemic steroids and theophylline.
- **Hypertension:** Bupropion has been reported to elevate blood pressure in patients with or without a previous history of hypertension.
- **Liver impairment**: Bupropion should be avoided in patients with liver cirrhosis and liver insufficiency.
- **Alcohol abuse**: Bupropion is not recommended in patient abusing alcohol.

- ➤ **Heart disease:** Bupropion need to be used with caution in patients with cardiac impairment.
- ➤ **Kidney impairment**: Bupropion should be used with caution in patients with renal impairment. A reduced dose is needed as bupropion and its metabolites may accumulate in the plasma to a greater extent.
- ➤ **Elderly:** Bupropion needs a dose in the elderly.

- ➤ **MAOI:** Bupropion requires **7- days** washout period before starting with MAOI. Bupropion requires a **3 weeks** washout period after MAOI was stopped before starting bupropion. Bupropion combined with MAOI may be fatal.

- ➤ **Thioridazine:** Buproprion combined with thioridazine must be avoided due to the increased risk of cardiac arrhythmias.
- ➤ **Anorexia:** Bupropion should be avoided in patients with anorexia nervosa.

Bupropion overdose

General symptoms of bupropion overdose

Initially, the patient might feel extremely tired and lethargic. The pulse will slow down, and the breathing frequency will also decrease. As the level of intoxication increases, the level of consciousness will decrease, and the patient will become unresponsive to external stimulations. The reflexes will disappear, and the breathing will get shallow. The patient's pulse and blood pressure will decrease until the cardiovascular system collapse.

Bupropion is **relatively safe in monotherapy overdoses** and has a rare incidence of fatalities. However, the concomitant use of bupropion with alcohol and with other central nervous depressants such as painkillers or benzodiazepines may result in a death cause by respiratory depression.

Seizure was reported to develop in up to 30% of overdose cases. Other prominent symptoms of overdose include hallucinations, loss of consciousness, sinus tachycardia, ECG changes, such as conduction disturbances, QRS prolongation, and arrhythmias. Bupropion overdose-related fatalities are attributed to large quantity of bupropion, which can cause uncontrolled seizures, bradycardia, cardiac failure and cardiac arrest.

General symptoms of bupropion over dose are

- **Seizure**
- **abnormal heart rhythm: tachycardia or bradycardia**
- **hallucinations**
- cardiac failure
- vomiting
- over sedation
- agitation
- loss of consciousness

What to do in the case of overdose

In general, there is no antidote for bupropion overdose. The management is mainly supportive which is aimed to maintain respiration, pulse and blood pressure.

In the event of a recent overdose with bupropion, a stomach washout, possibly with activated charcoal, may help to eliminate the un- absorbed drug and is done with large – bore oro-gastric tube, maintaining appropriate airway protection.

In some ER departments ipecac is also used in order to induce vomiting of the ingested toxin, however **induction of emesis is not recommended in semi-comatose and comatose patients**.

Due to the bupropion's large volume of distribution, forced diuresis, dialysis hemo- perfusion and exchange transfusion are unlikely to be effective.

Keeping open the patient's airway is compulsory, especially in semi - comatose individuals. The patient should be placed at his side in order to prevent respiration of the vomitus back to the lungs.

Suffocation due to vomit is the leading cause of death in bupropion overdose. Blood pressure and heart rate monitoring is very important. Fluid intake should be monitored with intra venous infusion of saline and urinary output should be also carefully monitored. In most cases, bupropion overdose, requires to hospitalize the patient for at least 24 hours for intense observation.

Bupropion references

1. Eric J NestlerHyman S, Malenka, R. Moleculat neuropharmacology. A foundation for clinical neuroscience. Mcgraw Hill companies, Inc. 2001.

2. Akamine, Yumiko,Yasui-Furukori et al. Psychotropic drug – drug interactions involving P-gp. 2012 Nov 2012 Vol 26 issue 11- 959 – 973.

3. Weiss j, Dormann SM, Martin- Facklam et al. Inhibition of P-gp by newer antidepressants. J. Pharmacol Exp Ther. 2003 Apr; 305(1):197-204.

4. Zung WWK, Brodie HKH, Fabre L et al.: Comparative efficacy and safety of bupropion and placebo in the

treatment of depression. Psychopharmacology (Berl) 1983,79:343-347.

7

Citalopram

Brand name: Cipramil, Celexa

Citalopram mode of action

Citalopram is a Serotonin Re Uptake

Transporter (SERT) <u>antagonist</u>: The inhibition of the Serotonin Reuptake Transporter (SERT) located on the presynaptic neurons, by citalopram, results in increased cortical serotonin levels.

In the SSRIs class, citalopram is one of the most selective inhibitor of the SERTs. In vivo, 20mg of citalopram are capable of occupying 77% of SERT's suggesting that the citalopram start dose of 20mg is adequate to produce the clinically significant antidepressant response.

The selective effects of citalopram on the anticholinergic, histaminergic and α adrenergic receptor are summarized as follows:

- ✓ **Anticholinergic Ach muscarinic affinity:** Low. Citalopram has low side effects symptoms of dry mouth, constipation, blurred vision and drowsiness.

- ✓ **Histaminergic H1 affinity:** Low. Citalopram has low side effects symptoms of sedation and weight gain.

- ✓ **α 1 adrenergic affinity:** Low. Citalopram has low side effect symptoms of hypotension, dizziness, drowsiness and other cardiovascular effects.

Pharmacokinetiks (PK) of citalopram

Citalopram & S-citalopram display **linear pharmacokinetics.** Both drugs apparently are able to inhibit their own metabolism. A dose increase of citalopram and S-citalopram will lead to a proportionate increase in their plasma levels. The overall pharmacokinetic profile of S-citalopram is very similar to that of citalopram.

Peak plasma level time (Tmax): 2 - 4 hours.

Steady state: Daily use of citalopram will result in a steady plasma level **within 7 days** of treatment and is often associated with significant reduction in side effects.

Absorption: Citalopram is well absorbed by the gastrointestinal system, and its absorption is **not** affected by the presence of food.

Protein binding: **80%**. Citalopram is mainly bound to albumin. The S- citalopram protein binding is only **56%**.

Half-life (T1/2): Citalopram 35 hours.

S- citalopram 27 – 32 hours

It appears that the citalopram half-life may be increased by 50% in patients above 60 years of age. There was no gender difference in citalopram steady state plasma levels, thus no dose adjustment is needed on the basis of gender.

Metabolism: Liver: CYP 450 iso-enzymes

        Citalopram: **2C19, 3A4 and 2D6**

        S-Citalopram: 2C19, 3A4

Citalopram is primarily metabolized by the liver by the iso-enzyme CYP450: **2C19, 3A4 and 2D6** to *demethylcitalopram* **(DCT)**, to *didemethylcitalopram* **(DDCT)**, and to *citalopram – N- oxide* as well as to a *deaminated propionic acid derivative*. **Citalopram metabolites are inactive** and have a plasma concentration of only 50% of that of the parent drug and a half-life of 50 hours.

Although the citalopram metabolite DCT has a very weak antagonistic action on the SERT, it has an 11-fold more inhibitory potency on the NET than that of its parent drug. However, due to its limited ability to cross the blood-brain barrier, citalopram metabolites have limited clinical relevance.

Patients with liver disease as well as elderly may experience a significant decrease in citalopram & S-Citalopram metabolism, which may result in higher citalopram blood levels and increased side effects. Therefore, patients with compromised liver require lower citalopram doses, which should be in the range of 10 – 20 mg a day in order to avoid excessive accumulation of the drug in the blood.

The P-gp System

Citalopram is a weak inhibitor of the P-gp functions in vivo and in vitro (1).

The inhibitory effects of citalopram on the P-gp system might interfere with the plasma levels of other co-administered drugs, which are also P-gp substrates. Furthermore, the P-gp system, which is present in the blood-brain-barrier (BBB) may play an important role in limiting the brain entry of citalopram as well as that of paroxetine, amitriptyline, venlafaxine, doxepin, and trimipramine (3).

Elimination : Citalopram is eliminated mainly by the **faeces**.

Patients with mild to moderate renal function impairment may experience reduced clearance of citalopram by 17% compared to normal patients.

How supplied

Citalopram

- Tablet: 10mg, 20mg, 40mg
- Capsules 10mg, 20mg, 40 mg

S-citalopram

- Tablet 5mg,10mg,20mg
- Capsules 5 mg, 10 mg, 20mg. oral solution 5mg/5ml.

Dose range

- 10mg – 50 mg for depression

Clinical indications: for citalopram and s – citalopram

- Major Depression(MDD)
- Panic disorder (PD)
- Obsessive compulsive disorder (OCD)
- Premenstrual dysphoric syndrome (PMDD)
- Post Traumatic Stress Disorder (PTSD)
- Generalised anxiety disorder (GAD)
- Social anxiety disorder (SAD)

Major Depression (MDD)

Several studies have established the superiority of citalopram & that of S-Citalopram over placebo in the treatment of major depression.

However, within the SSRI class, there is no evidence for superior effectiveness of one SSRI over another. In addition, there is no direct relationship between citalopram plasma concentrations and the clinical response. Furthermore, both citalopram and S-citalopram have been shown to have a long term efficacy, and could prevent depressive relapses during long-term use.

The effectiveness of citalopram in the real world was evaluated in the Sequenced Treatment Alternatives to Relieve Depression (STAR*D) published in 2006, it involved 2876 outpatients from 23 psychiatric and 18 primary care setting. All patients received citalopram with a mean dose of 40mg/day for up to 14 weeks.

The response rate was measured by self- report, using the 16-items QIDS-SR and defined as a >50% symptom reduction from baseline. On the QIDS-SR, remission was defined as a score of <5. The primary outcome measure was the 17-item HAMD rating scale and defined as an exit score of <7 for remission.

The SRAR*D study citalopram response and remission rates are illustrated in figure 7.1.

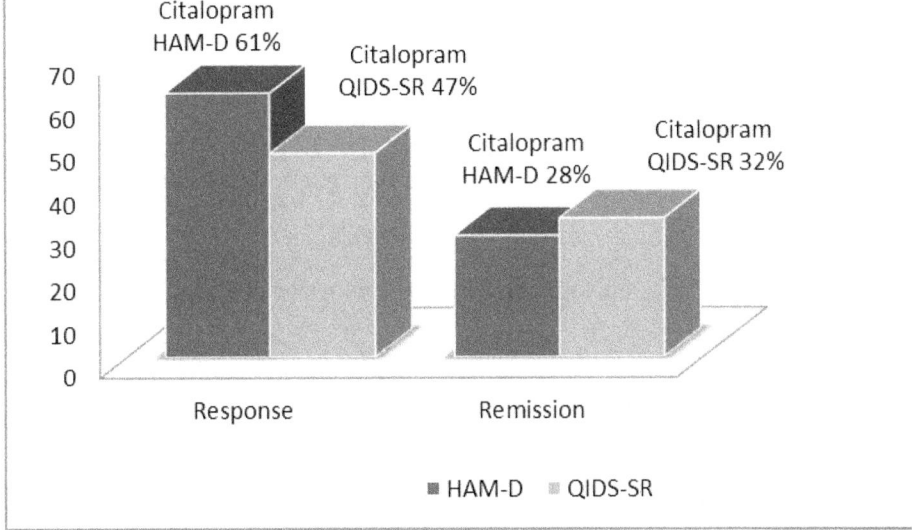

Figure 7.1: STAR*D: Results of citalopram HAM-D and QIDS-SR remission and response rates in the 2.876 outpatients with MDD. Response defined as >50% improvement from baseline on the Hamilton Rating scale for depression (HAM-D) and Remission defined as HAM-D score of <7 after 14 weeks of treatment. Adapted from Trivedi M, Rush AJ, Wisniewski SR et al. Evaluation of outcome with citalopram for depression using measurement – based care in STAR*D: implications for clinical practice. Am J Psychiatry Januarry 2006; 163:1.

OCD

Citalopram and S- citalopram have been shown to have significant efficacy in the treatment of Obsessive-Compulsive Disorder (OCD) independent of the patient's mood. Citalopram appeared to be effective in controlling both the obsessive and the compulsive component of the disorder.

Panic disorder (PD)

PD has a life time prevalence of 3.5% in the general population. Almost 30% of the patients with PD also experience comorbid depression.

Citalopram & S- citalopram were shown to be effective in the treatment of panic disorder in the acute phase as well as in long term use.

Post Traumatic Stress Disorder (PTSD)

Citalopram & S-citalopram were shown to be effective in the treatment of PTSD both in the acute phase as well as in long term use.

Premenstrual Dysphoric Disorder (PMDD)

PMDD affects up to 8% of the woman during their reproductive life. It is characterized by symptoms of bloating, weight gain, poor concentration, disturbed sleep, irritability, tension and depressed mood.

These symptoms get worse before the menses and often resolve upon menstruation. Both Citalopram & S-citalopram were effective in reducing the physical and the psychological symptoms of PMDD at doses of 10 - 20mg a day.

Social Anxiety Disorder

Citalopram & S-citalopram were shown to be effective in the treatment of Social anxiety disorder. The optimal daily dose of citalopram is 20mg.

Generalised Anxiety Disorder (GAD)

GAD is a common disorder with a lifetime prevalence of 3% in the general population. GAD characterized by persistent worry associated with poor concentration, muscle tension, sleep disturbances and tension headache. In addition, nearly 70% of the patient with GAD also experience a comorbid depression.

Citalopram & S-citalopram were shown to be effective in the treatment of the acute phase of GAD as well as in the long-term use at dose levels of 10 mg – 20 mg a day.

The effects of citalopram on the GAD symptoms can last up to 6 months after the treatment was terminated.

How to treat with citalopram and s-citalopram

Major Depression (MDD)

- **Citalopram:** Start with 20mg a day in a single morning dose. Wait at least two weeks to assess the clinical status before increasing the dose up to a maximum of 40mg a day. Citalopram can be administered in the morning or at night as a once-daily single dose.

- **S- citalopram**: Start with an initial dose of 10 mg of S-citalopram a day and increase up to 20 mg/day if needed. S-citalopram can be administered in the morning or at night as a daily single dose.

In general, 10 mg of s-citalopram is comparable to 40 mg of citalopram and appeared to have a fewer side effects.

Recently the FDA issued a warning for citalopram use to be limited to a maximum of 40 mg a day due to its ability to cause abnormal changes in the heart electrical activities such as QTC prolongation that can lead to cardiac arrhythmias.

It appears that the risk of cardiac arrhythmias is higher in predisposed patients who in addition have low blood levels of potassium (K) and magnesium (Mg) in their blood.

For the treatment of OCD

The average dose of citalopram for the treatment of OCD is 40mg a day, and it requires at least 3-12 weeks of treatment before clinical improvement can be achieved.

For the treatment of PD

The treatment with citalopram should start with a lower dose, e.g., 5 mg a day, in order to avoid worsening of anxiety symptoms, a common clinical reaction to citalopram at the initial phase of the treatment. Gradual dose increase should be given as clinically required. Although the current available data suggest that the effective dose of citalopram is 20 mg a day, inter-individual variation shows that some individuals can benefit from lower doses.

The duration of treatment with citalopram for panic disorder is 6 – 12 months. However, in some cases a longer period of treatment is required in order to control PD symptoms and in some cases the treatment should continue indefinitely.

When and how to take citalopram

Citalopram & S-citalopram can be taken either in the morning or in the evening in a single daily dose.

How to stop citalopram

Due to their short half-life, and the possibility to develop withdrawal syndrome, upon abrupt discontinuation, a slow tapering off citalopram & S-Citalopram is strongly recommended.

Sudden discontinuation of citalopram may cause discontinuation symptoms due to citalopram's relative short half-life and the lack of therapeutic effect of its principal metabolites. The dose of citalopram should be reduced gradually by a 50% dose reduction every third day. In the case of a patient getting withdrawal symptoms, reinstate the previous dose, and once the symptoms disappear start reducing the citalopram dose more slowly and over longer period of time. In some cases, the addition of another SSRI which has a longer half-life (such as fluoxetine) can be used in order to minimize the emergence of withdrawal symptoms.

How long it takes to get an antidepressant effect

In order to get an antidepressant effect, citalopram and S-citalopram should be used daily for at least 2 – 4 weeks. In some cases, dose increase might lead to a better clinical response. Like all antidepressants, both citalopram and S-citalopram requires time before a substantial mood improvement can be evident.

Side effects of citalopram

Citalopram side effects are dose related and tend to emerge when the drug reaches its peak plasma level. A single dose of citalopram may cause side effects within the first 2-4 hours of drug ingestion.

Citalopram side effects are probably related to its effects on the serotonin levels in the brain and other body parts. Side effects normally develop soon after the initiation of treatment with citalopram and often disappear with time. The side effects associated with S-citalopram are similar to those observed with citalopram.

The most common side effects of citalopram are:

Nervous system:

- insomnia
- agitation,
- restlessness, jitteriness anxiety

- tremor
- increased sweating/ flushing
- headache
- dizziness
- seizures (rare)
- somnolence
- sedation
- fatigue
- cognitive slowing
- reduced attention
- apathy
- emotional blunting
- rash

Gastro intestinal: The GI side effects are common with citalopram and usually develop within 30 minutes of citalopram ingestion.

The GI side effects are more likely the result of the direct effect of citalopram on the intestinal mucosa. The most common GI adverse effects are:

- decreased appetite upper gastrointestinal symptoms
- nausea,
- vomiting,
- dry mouth
- diarrhea
- constipation
- possible weight loss

Sexual : The incidence of the sexual side effects with SSRIs use develops in 20 % - 40% of treated patients. Citalopram sexual side effects are dose dependent and do not diminish over time.

However, most of the citalopram sexual side effects disappear upon treatment discontinuation.

The most common citalopram sexual side effects are:

- decreased sex drive
- delayed ejaculation
- impotence
- inability to reach an orgasm

Suicide

The FDA requires all antidepressants to carry a black box warning stating that antidepressant may increase the risk for suicide in persons under the age of 25 years. This warning is based on data suggesting that suicidal ideations and behaviour has a 2 fold increase in children and in adolescents, and 1.5 – fold increase in the 18 – 24 age group.

Citalopram side effects that need immediate attention:

- Confusion
- Excitation
- Onset of seizure
- Yellow skin / eyes
- Severe allergic reaction
- Irregular heart beats Arrythmia
- Low blood pressure
- Bruising and bleeding (relatively rare)
- Induction of manic episode
- Activation of suicidal ideation and behaviour

Physical and psychological dependence

In animal studies, citalopram did not show abuse potential.

Furthermore, in human clinical trials, there was no indication of drug seeking behaviour, euphoria and drug liking. However, citalopram can cause physical dependence, as evidenced by the presence of withdrawal symptoms upon abrupt discontinuation of citalopram. Citalopram physical symptoms of dependence are similar to those of other SSRIs and SNRIs. In general, clinicians should carefully monitor the patients for signs of misuse or abuse.

Citalopram discontinuation symptoms are

- Electric shock sensation
- insomnia
- dizziness
- light-handedness
- vertigo
- irritability
- bladder control problems
- akathisia: inability to stand still -
- Anxiety

Safety profile of citalopram

Use in pregnancy: Risk category C

Citalopram is classified by the FDA as having a **risk category C**. The risk of pregnant mothers with a history of depression to develop depression during their pregnancy and especially after child delivery is very high and often requires the continuation of the treatment with SSRIs during and after the pregnancy.

In animal reproductive studies, citalopram was shown to have teratogenic effects when given at doses above human therapeutic range. In addition, in a pregnant rat study, oral administration of citalopram during the period of organogenesis resulted in decreased fetal growth and survival and increased incidence of cardiovascular and skeletal defects at doses of 18 times the

MRHD. There are no well-controlled studies in pregnant woman.

In addition, the use of citalopram in the last trimester of pregnancy is associated with higher incidence of respiratory distress and pulmonary hypertension, cyanosis, apnea, seizures, temperature instability vomiting, hypoglycaemia, hypotonia, hyperreflexia, tremor, irritability, constant crying and jitteriness which required prolonged hospitalization, tube feeding and respiratory support. There is an increased risk of the newborn developing PPHN, which is associated with substantial neonatal morbidity and mortality.

The risk of developing PPHN was six-fold higher in infants exposed to SSRIs after the 20th week of gestation. The risk of getting PPHN appeared to be common to all SSRIs. The effects of citalopram on labor and delivery is unknown. Therefore, the use of citalopram during the first trimester as well as throughout the pregnancy is not recommended, and risk versus benefits should be carefully discussed with the patient.

Use during lactation

Citalopram & S- citalopram are secreted in the breast milk. Excessive somnolence, decreased feeding and weight loss was observed in breastfeeding newborns in citalopram-treated mothers.

Due to unknown effects on the newborn's normal growth and development, breastfeeding should be avoided.

Citalopram drug interaction

- **Warfarin:** The concomitant use of citalopram with warfarin may Increased warfarin blood levels, which carry the risk of bleeding. Protrombin time was increased by 5%.

- **MAOI;** The concomitant use of citalopram with MAOI may lead to CNS toxicity and serotonin syndrome. The patient must wait 21 days after MAOI is stopped before initiating treatment with citalopram. After stopping citalopram, wait 7 days to start treatment with MAOI.
- **Metroprolol:** The concomitant use of citalopram with metroplolol may Increased metoprolol blood levels by 100%. When it is co-administered with S-citalopram metoprolol blood levels increase by 50%.
- **Pimozide & Thioridazine:** The concomitant use of citalopram with Pimozide & Thioridazine may Increased plasma levels of both antipsychotics medications which can cause cardiac arrhythmias.
- **Tramadol:** The concomitant use of citalopram with tramadol may cause seizures.
- **Sumatriptan :** The concomitant use of citalopram with sumatriptan may cause weakness and hyperreflexia and incoordination.
- **Carbamazepine:** The concomitant use of citalopram with carbamazepine may increase the clearance of citalopram.
- **Ketoconazole:** The concomitant use of citalopram with ketoconazole may decreased ketoconazole Cmax by 21%.

Warning for citalopram

> **Pregnancy: Risk category C.** Try to avoid the use during pregnancy or breastfeeding. Assessment of the risk versus benefits must be discussed with the patient.
> **Citalopram may cause an increase in suicidal risk in young adults.** Pooled analysis of trials of drugs used for MDD showed that SNRIs and SSRIs may increase the risk of suicidal thinking and behavior in children, adolescents and young adults aged 18-24. The use of antidepressants in this population must balance the risk of suicide with the

clinical need. Careful monitoring of the patient's clinical worsening, and suicidality should also involve the family and all other caregivers.

- **Serotonin syndrome** may develop with citalopram use. Serotonin syndrome symptoms may include agitation, dizziness, hallucinations, delirium, seizures and coma along with autonomic instability, which include tachycardia, fluctuating blood pressure, flushing, hyperthermia, tremor, muscular rigidity, myoclonus, hyperreflexia, and incoordination. The concomitant use of citalopram with MAOI, triptans, TCAs, Lithium, fentanyl, tramadol, tryptophan, buspirone and St. John Worth may precipitate serotonin syndrome.

- **Activation of hypomania or mania** occurred only in 0.2% of citalopram treated bipolar patients.

- **The incidence of seizures** occurrs in **0.3%** of citalopram treated patients.

- **Discontinuation response** may develop upon sudden discontinuation of citalopram. The most common discontinuation symptoms include dysphoric mood, agitation, anxiety, dizziness irritability, paresthesias in the form of electric shock sensations, headaches, insomnia, emotional lability, lethargy and confusion. A gradual dose reduction is strongly recommended.

- **Hyponatremia** may develop subsequent to the use of citalopram, especially in volume-depleted patients and in patients on diuretics. It is possible that hyponaremia results from the syndrome of inappropriate antidiuretic hormone secretion (SIADH). The symptoms of hyponatremia include headaches, reduced concentration, confusion, weakness and unsteadiness, which may lead to fall. Severe cases of hyponatremia may result in seizures, hallucination's respiratory arrest, coma and death. Elderly

patients appeared to be at a higher risk. Discontinuing citalopram often results in symptom resolution.
- **Angle – closure glaucoma**: Citalopram may have an effect on the pupil size resulting in mydriasis. Patients with narrow angle glaucoma may experience increased intraocular pressure when are treated with citalopram.
- **Abnormal bleeding** was observed in patients using citalopram. Concomitant use of warfarin, non steroidal anti- inflammatory drugs (NSAIDs) and aspirin may add to this risk.
- **Elderly**: Citalopram need a lower dose when it is used in patients above 60 years.
- **Liver impairment**: Citalopram needs a lower dose when it is used in patients with moderate liver impairment.
- **MAOI**: Citalopram may cause serotonin syndrome when it is used in combination with MAOIs. Citalopram users require at least 2 weeks of a washout period before starting with MAOI and 21 days of wash out period after MAOI discontinuation.

Citalopram Overdose:

Citalopram overdose can be either unintentional, or intentional. The effects of citalopram overdose also depend on whether it was ingested alone or in combination with other drugs or alcohol. As a general rule, the bigger the amount of citalopram ingested, the worse the reaction and the higher the possibilities for lethal results.

General symptoms of citalopram overdose:

Initially, the patient might feel extremely tired and lethargic. The pulse will slow down, and the breathing frequency will also decrease.

As the level of intoxication increases, the level of consciousness will decrease, and the patient will become unresponsive to external stimulations. The reflexes will disappear, and the breathing will get shallow. The patient's pulse and blood pressure will decrease until cardiovascular system collapse.

Citalopram & S-Citalopram are **rarely lethal in monotherapy overdose**. However, the concomitant use of citalopram with alcohol and/or with other central nervous depressants such as painkillers or benzodiazepines may result in death cause by respiratory depression.

The most common symptoms of citalopram over dose are:

- nausea
- vomiting
- over sedation
- somnolence
- agitation
- abnormal heart rhythm: sinus tachycardia
- QTc prolongation
- dizziness
- sweating
- tremor
- convulsions
- amnesia
- confusion
- seizures
- cyanosis
- rabdomyolysis
- coma

What to do in the case of citalopram overdose:

In general, there is no antidote for citalopram overdose and the management is mainly supportive which is aimed to maintain respiration, pulse and blood pressure. In the event of a recent overdose with citalopram, a stomach washout with activated charcoal might help in the elimination of the un- absorbed drug. In some ER departments, ipecac is also used in order to induce vomiting of the ingested toxin, however **induction of emesis is <u>not</u> recommended in semi-comatose and comatose patients**. Due to the large volume of distribution of citalopram, forced diuresis, dialysis hemo- perfusion and exchange transfusion are unlikely to be effective. Keeping open the patient's airway is compulsory, especially in that semi - comatose individuals.

The patient should be placed at his side in order to prevent respiration of the vomitus to the lungs. Suffocation due to vomit is the leading cause of death in citalopram overdose. Blood pressure and heart rate monitoring is very important. Fluid intake should be monitored with intra venous infusion of saline and urinary output should be also carefully monitored. In most cases, citalopram overdose, requires hospitalization for at least 24 hours for intense observation.

Citalopram references

1 Weiss j, Dormann SM, Martin- Facklam et al. Inhibition of P-gp by newer antidepressants. J. Pharmacol Exp Ther. Apr 2003; 305(1):197-204.

2 Akamine, Yumiko,Yasui-Furukori et al. Psychotropic drug – drug interactions involving P-gp. Nov 2012 Vol 26 issue 11- 959 – 973.

3 Jun-Sheng W, Hao-Jie Z. Bryan BG et al. Sertraline and its metabolite desmethylsertraline, but not Buprorion or its three major metabolites, have high affinity for P-gp. Biol Pharm Bull Feb 2008: 31(2): 231 – 234.

4 Trivedi M, Rush AJ, Wisniewski SR et al. Evaluation of outcome with citalopram for depression using measurement – based care in STAR*D: implications for clinical practice. Am J Psychiatry Januarry 2006;163:1.

8

Clomipramine

Brand name: Anafranil,

Generic: Clomidep, Equinorm

Mode of action: Clomipramine

1. Clomipramine is a potent antagonist of the serotonin reuptake transporter (SERT): The inhibition of the SERT, located on the presynaptic neurons, by clomipramine, results in increased serotonin synaptic levels. It appears that the inhibition of SERT by clomipramine is as strong as that of the other SSRIs.

1. **Desmethylclomipramine (DMI), which is clomipramine's active metabolite, is a strong antagonist of the norepinephrine reuptake transporter (NET):** The inhibition of the presynaptic NET results in increased norepinephrine synaptic levels.

The selective effects of clomipramine on the anticholinergic, histaminergic and α adrenergic receptors are summarized as follows:

- ✓ **Anticholinergic Ach muscarinic affinity: High.** Clomipramine use may cause severe anticholinergic side effects which includes dry mouth, constipation, blurred vision and drowsiness.

- ✓ **Histaminergic H1 affinity: Moderate.** Clomipramine use may cause moderate histaminergic side effects which include sedation and weight gain.

✓ **α 1 adrenergic affinity: High.** Clomipramine use may cause severe adrenergic related side effects which include hypotension, dizziness, drowsiness and other cardiovascular effects

Pharmacokinetics of Clomipramine

Clomipramine has **linear pharmacokinetics.** Thus, any dose change leads to a proportional change in the drug plasma levels.

Peak plasma levels (Tmax): 2 – 6 hours

As clomipramine side effects are dose-related and tend to emerge at the peak of its plasma level, a single dosing of clomipramine may result in emerging side effects within 2 hours after drug ingestion.

Absorption: Clomipramine is well absorbed by the gastrointestinal system and **it is not affected by the presence of food in the stomach.**

Protein bounding: 98%. Clomipramine is highly protein bounded mainly to albumin and α1glycoprotein.

Half- life (T1/2): 32 hours for the parent drug.

69 hours for the active metabolite (DMI).

Clomipramine's active metabolite *Desmethylclomipramine* **(DMI)** has an affinity for the presynaptic norepinephrine transporter (NET). The longer half-life of *desmethylclomipramine* **(DMI)** results in a reduced risk for discontinuation symptoms and a higher risk of drug interaction.

Bioavailability 50%

Steady state: Clomipramine reach a steady state concentration within **7-14 days** of regular use. Clomipramine is highly lipophilic and tend to concentrate in high levels in the brain and in the cardiac tissue.

Metabolism: Clomipramine is primarily metabolized by the liver via the enzyme CYP450: **2D6 and 1A2.**

The P-gp System

Clomipramine **is not a P-gp substrate** and it is not significantly affected by the P-gp system (3).

Elimination: Urine 60%, Faeces 30%

How supplied

- Clomipramine capsules of 25mg, 50mg, 75mg
- Clomipramine CR 75 mg.

Dose range

- Clomipramine 100 mg – 200mg a day for depression
- Clomipramine CR 75mg – 150mg a day for depression

Clomipramine Clinical indications

- Major depression
- Treatment resistant depression
- Anxiety
- Neuropathic pain
- Premature ejaculation
- Enuresis (involuntary nightly urination during sleep) in children and adolescents.
- Cataplexy syndrome

Major Depressive Disorder (MDD)

Clomipramine showed comparable efficacy to that of other tricyclic antidepressants in the treatment of MDD. Early studies showed clomipramine has a 65% efficacy rates for the treatment of depression as compared to a 30% improvement with placebo.

In a double-blind study of the efficacy and safety of sertraline and clomipramine in 166 outpatients with severe MDD for 8 weeks, 74% of sertraline group patients and 71% of the clomipramine group responded to treatment as measured by 17-items HAM-D. The HAM-D scores fell from 29.8 at baseline to 12.3 at the endpoint in the sertraline group, and from 29.6 to 12.7 in the clomipramine group (4).

Long term effects of clomipramine were studied by the Danish university antidepressant group. In this studies (6,7) clomipramine showed better remission rates than those of citalopram and paroxetine. Although the FDA approved the use of clomipramine only for the treatment of OCD, in Europe clomipramine is regarded as one of the most potent and effective antidepressants.

Follows in Figure 8.1 clomipramine response and remission rates studies.

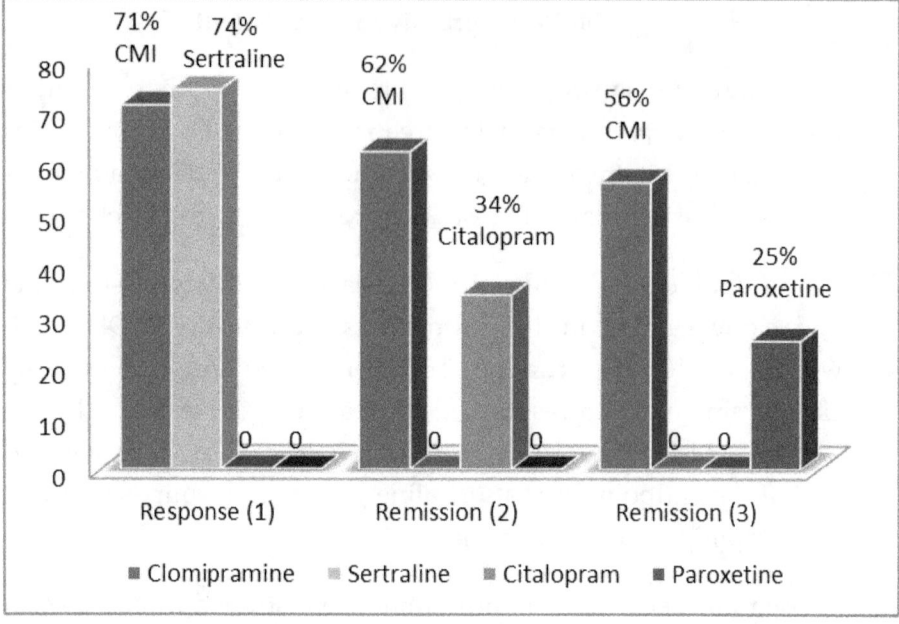

Figure 8.1 Clomipramine (CMI) and sertraline response rates in the treatment of MDD. Response defined as >50% improvement from baseline in the Hamilton Rating scale for depression (HAM-D) and Remission defined as HAM-D score of <6 after 8 weeks of treatment. Adapted from Lepine JP, Goger J, Blashko C. A double blind study of the efficacy and safety of sertraline and clomipramine in outpatients with severe MDD. Int Clin Psychoparmacol 2000 Sep.; 15(5):263-271.

2. **Clomipramine (CMI) and citalopram remission rates in the treatment of MDD.** Adapted from the Danish university antidepressant group. Citalopram clinical effect profile in comparison with clomipramine. A controlled multicentre study. Psychopharmacology, 1986, 90, 131-138.

3. **Clomipramine(CMI) and paroxetine remission rates in the treatment of MDD.** Adapted from the Danish university

antidepressant group. Comparative efficacy of clomipramine versus paroxetine in endogenous MDD. Journal of Affective Disorders, 1990,18,289-299.

Obsessive compulsive disorder (OCD)

Among the TCA medications, clomipramine is the strongest inhibitor of the serotonin reuptake transporter (SERT) which makes it an effective drug for the treatment of OCD. In a single-blind 12 weeks controlled study of Venlafaxine versus clomipramine in the treatment of OCD, both drugs showed similar response rates, with 34.6% for venlafaxine treated patients and 42.6% for the clomipramine-treated patients (5).

The results of this study are illustrated in Figure 8.2

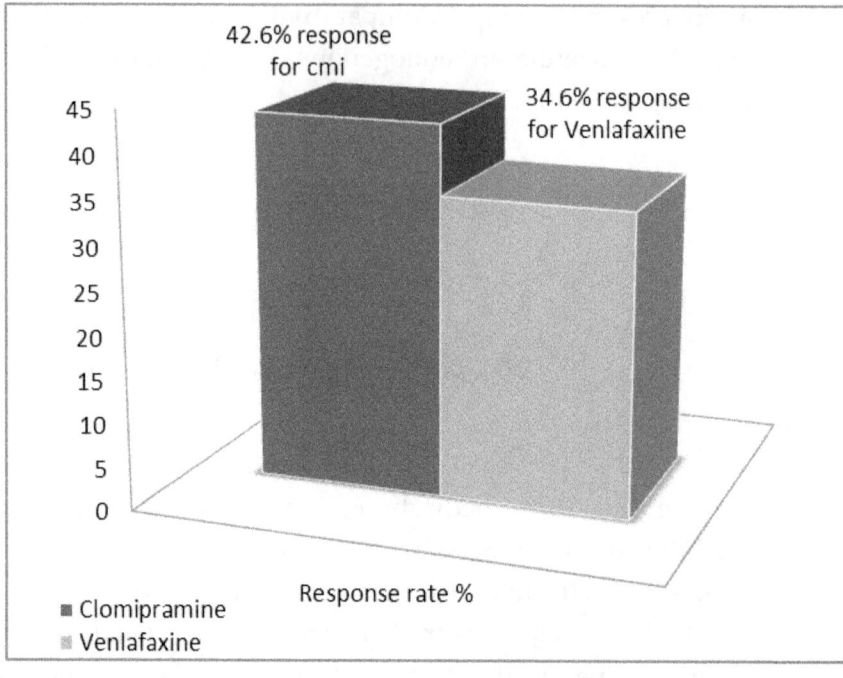

Figure 8.2 Clomipramine(CMI) and venlafaxine response rates in the treatment of OCD. Response defined as >50% improvement from baseline. Adapted from Albert V, Aguglia E, Maina G. Venlafaxine versus clomipramine in the treatment of OCD. A preliminary single-blind 12 weeks controlled study. J Clin Psychiatry, Nov 2002;63(11):1004-1011.

There is the suggestion that clomipramine is even more effective than the SSRIs for the treatment of OCD.

Enuresis & premature ejaculation

Clomipramine, like other TCAs, is highly effective in preventing involuntary night-time urination during sleep as well as in delaying ejaculation during sexual intercourse. It is believed that the anticholinergic side effect of clomipramine are responsible for the beneficial effects in these two conditions.

How to treat with clomipramine

For Major Depression (MDD): Start with clomipramine 25mg, preferably at bedtime, and slowly increase the dose by increments of 25mg every 3 days up to a maximum of 200mg taken at bedtime in order to avoid excessive daily sedation.

For OCD: Start with clomipramine 25mg once a day at bedtime to be increased every 3 days by increments of 25 mg up to a maximum dose of 250mg.

When and how to take medication

Preferably take clomipramine at bedtime to avoid over-sedation. In general, "start low and go slow" as patients can experience over sedation the following day at the beginning of the treatment.

How to stop clomipramine

It is highly recommended to slowly taper clomipramine in order to minimize the emergence of withdrawal symptoms, which usually develops within the first 2 weeks of treatment cessation.

Clomipramine requires a 50% dose reduction every third day.

In the event of the patient developing withdrawal symptoms, reinstate the previous dose and once the symptoms disappear, start reducing the clomipramine dose in smaller increments and over longer period of time.

How long it takes to get an antidepressant effect

Like all antidepressants, clomipramine needs at least 7 – 28 days before a substantial mood improvement emerges

Side effects of clomipramine

Most side effects of clomipramine are probably related to its ability to increase serotonin in the brain, as well as its inhibitory effects on the α1 adrenergic receptors, the H1 histaminergic receptors and the anticholinergic muscarinic receptors. The inhibition of α1 adrenergic receptors may results in hypotension while the inhibition of H1 receptors may result in oversedation and weight gain. Most side effects of clomipramine are dose-related and often develop soon after the initiation of treatment and subside with time. The most common side effects of clomipramine are:

Nervous system

- drowsiness
- lethargy
- fatigue
- weakness
- dizziness
- insomnia
- nausea
- blurred vision
- headache and worsening of migraine
- In coordination
- tremor
- disturbed concentration
- disorientation
- confusion
- restlessness and agitation (rare)
- *seizures* (clomipramine has the highest incidence among all TCAs to cause seizures especially in predisposed individuals. The incidence of seizure in patients on clomipramine is 2% at doses above 300mg a day.
- stuttering

- disturbance in gait
- worsening of parkinsonism
- rash (rare)

Cardiac
- hypotension
- syncope
- bradycardia

Gastro intestinal:

The gastro intestinal side effects can develop within 30 minutes of drug ingestion, and they are more likely the result of clomipramine anticholinergic effects.

- *decreased appetite*
- *heartburn*
- **weight gain (in 18% of patients)**
- nausea
- vomiting
- dry mouth
- constipation
- gastritis

Sexual
- decreased libido
- Impotence
- retrograde ejaculation
- painful ejaculation
- delayed ejaculation

Practical implication: due to its strong anticholinergic effects, clomipramine can be used for the treatment of premature ejaculation.

Suicide

The FDA requires all antidepressants to carry a black box warning stating that antidepressants may increase the risk for suicide in persons under the age of 25 years. This warning is based on data suggesting that suicide ideations and behavior has a 2-fold increase in children and in adolescents, and 1.5 – fold increase in the 18 – 24 age group.

Clomipramine Side effect that requires immediate attention

- Confusion
- Excitation
- Onset of seizure
- Yellow skin /eye
- Severe allergic reaction
- Irregular heart beats
- Hypotension
- Induction of manic or hypomanic episode
- Activation of suicidal ideation and behaviour especially in children and adolescents

Physical & psychological dependence

Patients treated with clomipramine did not show any tendencies for drug seeking behaviour. However, patients with a history of drug abuse should be closely monitored for signs of clomipramine misuse or abuse, which include drug seeking behavior, development of tolerance and dose increase.

Clomipramine discontinuation reaction

A sudden discontinuation of clomipramine may be associated with a discontinuation reaction. The discontinuation symptoms are usually self-limiting. The most common symptoms of clomipramine discontinuation reaction are:

- irritability
- agitation
- dizziness
- anxiety
- confusion
- headache
- lethargy
- insomnia
- seizures
- dysphoric mood
- fever
- fatigue
- sweating
- myalgia (muscle pain)

A slow down titration of clomipramine is often associated with a reduced risk of having the discontinuation reaction

Safety profile of clomipramine

Use in pregnancy: FDA risk category C

According the FDA, clomipramine has a **risk category C**. The risk of pregnant mothers with a history of depression to develop depression during their pregnancy and especially after child delivery is very high and often requires the continuation of the treatment with SSRIs during and after the pregnancy. No teratogenic effects were seen in studies performed in rats at doses of 24 times of the maximum human dose (MRHD).

However, the use of clomipramine in the last trimester of pregnancy is associated with higher incidence of respiratory distress and pulmonary hypertension, cyanosis, apnea, seizures, temperature instability vomiting, hypoglycemia, hypotonia, hyperreflexia, tremor, irritability, constant crying and jitteriness, which required prolonged hospitalization, tube feeding and respiratory support.

There is an increased risk of the newborn to develop Persistent Pulmonary Hypertension of the Newborn (PPHN), and it is associated with substantial neonatal morbidity and mortality. In general, the risk of developing PPHN was six-fold higher in infants exposed to SSRIs after the 20th week of gestation. It appears that the risk of getting PPHN is common to all antidepressants used during the pregnancy. Thus, the use of clomipramine during the first trimester as well as throughout the pregnancy is not recommended.

Use during lactation

Clomipramine is secreted in the breast milk. Due to its unknown effects on the newborn's normal growth and development, breast feeding should be avoided in a mother using clomipramine.

Carcinogenesis

There is no evidence of carcinogenesis, teratogenicity, mutagenicity or impaired fertility with clomipramine use.

Treatment of mice and rats with doses of 20 times the maximum recommended human dose (MRHD) showed no evidence of carcinogenicity.

Additionally, treatment of rats at doses 6 times the maximum recommended human dose showed no effects on fertility.

Avoid using clomipramine in the following cases

- **Myocardial infraction**: patients recovering from myocardial infraction should avoid using clomipramine due to its propensity to cause cardiac arrhythmias, prolongation of conduction time and hypotension.

- **Hyperthyroidism:** Patients with hyper active thyroid gland are more sensitive to the clomipramine side effects.
- **Cardiac arrhythmia:** Patients with pre-existing cardiac disease and cardiac arrhythmias should be closely monitored and preferably avoid the use of clomipramine.
- **History of seizure**
- **Prostate hypertrophy**
- **Pre-existing closed angle glaucoma**
- **Proven allergy to clomipramine**

Clomipramine drug interaction

Clomipramine Drug interactions are due to its metabolism by the liver enzyme CYP 450: **3A4** and **2D6**. Follows a list of clomipramine drug interactions with the possible clinical consequences.

- **Tramadol:** May increase the risk of seizure.
- **Warfarin:** May increased PT Time.
- **Carbamazepine:** May Decreased clomipramine plasma levels due to the P450 liver enzyme induction caused by carbamazepine.
- **Antiarrhytmic:** May cause Prolongation of cardiac conduction.
- **Phenobarbital:** May increase phenobarbital plasma level.
- **Akineton:** May increase clomipramine anticholinergic effect.
- **Fluoxetine:** May increase clomipramine plasma levels.
- **Ketoconazole:** May increase clomipramine plasma levels.
- **MAOI:** May cause CNS toxicity and serotonin syndrome. Wait 21 days after MAOI was stopped before initiating treatment with clomipramine. Wait 5-7 days to start MAOI after discontinuing clomipramine.
- **Methylphenidate:** May increase clomipramine plasma levels.

- **Cimetidine:** May cause increased clomipramine plasma concentration.
- **Fluvoxamine:** May increase clomipramine plasma concentration.
- **Grapefruit juice:** May decrease clomipramine metabolism due to inhibition of the liver enzyme **3A4**.
- **Tamoxifen:** May decrease clomipramine plasma levels.
- **Triptan:** May cause serotonergic reaction.

Warning for clomipramine

➢ **Pregnancy: Risk category** C. Try to avoid use during pregnancy or breastfeeding. Assessment of the risks versus benefits must be discussed with the patient

➢ **Seizure risk.** Clomipramine doses higher than 250mg are associated with an increased risk of seizure. The incidence of seizure in patients on clomipramine at doses of 300mg was 1.5%. Caution should be used when clomipramine is given to patients with a history of seizure and to patients who are predisposed to develop seizures such as known epileptics and patients with brain damage, as well as alcohol abusers.

➢ **Clomipramine may cause an increase in suicidal risk in young adults.** Pooled analysis of trials of drugs used for MDD showed that SNRIs and SSRIs may increase the risk of suicidal thinking and behavior in children, adolescents and young adults aged 18-24. In general, the use of antidepressants in this population must balance the risk of suicide with the clinical need. Careful monitoring of the patient's clinical worsening, and suicidality should also involve the family and all other caregivers..

➢ **Activation of hypomania or mania** may occurred in clomipramine treated bipolar patients. As clomipramine may trigger mania in the predisposed patients, it should be

used cautiously in patients with a history of bipolar mood disorder.
- **Serotonin syndrome** may develop with clomipramine use. Serotonin syndrome symptoms may include agitation, dizziness, hallucinations, delirium, seizures and coma along with autonomic instability which include tachycarfia, fluctuating blood pressure, flushing, hyperthermia, tremor, muscular rigidity, myoclonus, hyperreflexia, and incoordination. The concomitant use of clomipramine with MAOI, triptans, TCA, Lithium, fentanyl, tramadol, tryptophan, buspirone and St. John's Worth may precipitate serotonin syndrome.
- **Cardiac impairment** clomipramine need to be used with caution in patients with cardiac impairment. Clomipramine use was associated with low blood pressure in 20% of patients. ECG abnormalities developed in 1.5% of patients using clomipramine and included ST-T wave changes, PVCs and intra- ventricular conduction abnormalities.
- **Status post MI**: Clomipramine should be avoided in a patient with a recent myocardial infarct.
- **Renal impairment**: Clomipramine requires a dose adjustment (lower dose) in patients with mild to moderate renal impairment.
- **Liver impairment**: Clomipramine must be avoided in patients with liver insufficiency. Clomipramine was associated with SGOT and SGPT elevation 3 times greater than the normal upper limit in up to 3% of treated patients. Rare reports of fatal liver injury have been associated with clomipramine use.
- **Alcohol:** Clomipramine is not recommended in patient using alcohol.
- **Withdrawal reaction.** Clomipramine may cause withdrawal reaction, which requires a slow reduction of

clomipramine doses. The onset of withdrawal symptoms is attributed to the clomipramine short half-life. Clomipramine withdrawal can develop as early as the second day after drug discontinuation and may persist for several days. The most common symptoms of clomipramine withdrawal are nausea, dizziness, insomnia, anxiety, tension and headache.

- **Narrow angel glaucoma**: Clomipramine use in patients with glaucoma may be associated with increased intraocular pressure due to it anticholinergic properties.
- **Urinary retention**: Clomipramine may worsen urinary retention in predisposed patients due to its anticholinergic properties.
- **Hyperthyroidism:** Clomipramine cardiac toxicity may be increased in patients with hyperthyroidism or in patients on thyroid medications.
- **Adrenal medulla tumours:** Clomipramine use in patients with adrenal tumours such as pheochromocytoma or neuroblastoma may be associated with hypertensive crisis.
- **MAOI:** Clomipramine combined with MAOI may be fatal. Clomipramine requires a **7 day** washout period before starting with MAOI. Initiating treatment with clomipramine after MAOI requires a **3 week** washout period after MAOI was stopped.
- **Elderly**: Clomipramine requires a lower dose in the elderly.
- **Weight**: Clomipramine may cause weight gain in **18%** of patients compared to 1% of patients receiving placebo.
- **Hematologic changes**: Clomipramine may be associated with leukopenia, agranulocytosis, thrombocytopenia, anemia, and pancytopenia. Leukocyte and differential blood count should be obtained in patients treated with clomipramine who develop fever and sore throat.

> **Hyperthermia**: Clomipramine was associated with hyperthermia especially when it was used in combination with other serotoninergic drugs.

Clomipramine overdose

The effects of clomipramine overdose depends on whether it was ingested alone or as a combination with other drugs or with alcohol.

Clomipramine may be lethal in monotherapy overdose.

As a general rule, the bigger the amount of clomipramine ingested, the worse the reaction will get and the higher the possibility for lethal results. One death occurred in a patient suspected of ingesting a dose of 7000mg of clomipramine. The lowest dose associated with a fatality was 750mg.

General symptoms of clomipramine overdose

Initially, the patient might feel extremely tired and lethargic. The pulse will slow down, and the breathing frequency will decreased. As the level of intoxication increases, the level of consciousness will decrease, and the patient will become unresponsive to external stimulations.

The reflexes will disappear, and the breathing will get shallow. The patient's pulse and blood pressure will drop until the cardiovascular system collapse

In addition, the concomitant use of clomipramine with alcohol and with other central nervous depressants such as painkillers or benzodiazepines may result in death cause by respiratory depression, cardio-respiratory arrest. Patient developing status epilepticus, metabolic acidosis and hypoxia may also lead to death.

Symptoms of clomipramine over dose are

- over sedation
- drowsiness
- respiratory depression
- cyanosis
- respiratory arrest
- seizure
- abnormal heart rhythm – mainly tachycardia
- ECG changes – particularly in QRS axis
- congestive heart failure
- cardiac arrest
- hypotension
- hyperactive reflexes
- muscle rigidity
- coreiform movements
- mydriasis
- oliguria
- anuria
- vomiting
- delirium
- loss of consciousness

What to do in the case of clomipramine overdose

In general, there is no antidote for clomipramine overdose and the management is mainly supportive which is aimed to maintain respiration, pulse and blood pressure.

In the event of a recent overdose with clomipramine a stomach washout possibly with activated charcoal might help in the elimination of the unabsorbed drug and is done with a large bore oro-gastric tube with appropriate airway protection.

In some ER departments, ipecac is also used in order to induce vomiting of the ingested toxin, however **induction of emesis is not recommended in semi-comatose and comatose patients**. Due to the large volume of distribution of clomipramine, forced diuresis, dialysis hemo- perfusion and exchange transfusion are unlikely to be effective. Keeping open the patient's airway is compulsory, especially in semi - comatose individuals.

The patient should be placed on his side in order to prevent respiration of the vomitus back to the lungs. Suffocation due to vomit is the leading cause of death in clomipramine overdose. Blood pressure and heart rate monitoring is very important. Increase fluid intake by intra venous infusion of saline and monitor urinary output.

In most cases, clomipramine overdose requires hospitalization of the patient for at least 24 hours for intense observation

Clomipramine references

1 Akamine, Yumiko,Yasui-Furukori et al. Psychotropic drug – drug interactions involving P-gp. Nov 2012 Vol 26 issue 11- 959 – 973.

2 Weiss j, Dormann SM, Martin- Facklam et al. Inhibition of P-gp by newer antidepressants. J. Pharmacol Exp Ther. Apr 2003; 305(1):197-204.

3 Bikadi Z, Harai I, Malik D. Predicting P-gp mediated drug transport based on support vector mechanism. PLoSone. 2011:6(10):e 25815.

4 LepineJP, Goger J, Blashko C. A double blind study of the efficacy and safety of sertraline and clomipramine in outpatients with severe MDD> Int Clin Psychoparmacol 2000 Sep.; 15(5):263-271.

5 Albert V, Aguglia E, Maina G. Venlafaxine versus clomipramine in the treatment of OCD. A preliminary single-blind 12 weeks controlled study. J Clin Psychiatry, Nov 2002:63(11):1004-1011.

6 Danish university antidepressant group. Citalopram clinical effect profile in comparison with clomipramine. A controlled multicentre study. Psychopharmacology, 1986, 90, 131-138.

7 Danish university antidepressant group. Comparative efficacy of clomipramine versus paroxetine in endogenous MDD. Journal of Affective Disorders, 1990,18,289-299.

9

Desvenlafaxine

Brand name: Pristiq

Desvenlafaxine is an extended- release tablet, of the isolated major active metabolite of venlafaxine.

Mode of action of Desvenlafaxine

1. Desvenlafaxine is a Serotonin Re-uptake Transporter (SERT) Antagonist: The inhibitory effects of desvenlafaxine on SERT are *8-10 times stronger* than its effects on the norepinephrine reuptake transporter (NET).

2. Desvenlafaxine is a Norepinephrine Re-uptake Transporter (NET) antagonist. The NET, located on the pre-synaptic nerve cell, is responsible for pumping the excess synaptic norepinephrine back into the pre-synaptic nerve cell. Thus the inhibition of NET results in increased synaptic norepinephrine. It appears that desvenlafaxine's has a greater inhibitory effect on NET than the parent drug.

3. Desvenlafaxine is a Dopamine Reuptake Transporter (DAT) Antagonist: The DAT, located on the pre-synaptic nerve cell, is responsible for pumping the excess synaptic dopamine back into the pre synaptic nerve cell. Therefore, **the inhibition of DAT results in more synaptic dopamine.** The effect of desvnlafaxine on DAT occurs in the frontal cortex.

Note: The inhibition of the SERT, NET and DAT transporters is dose-dependent. At lower doses, desvenlafaxine, like the parent drug venlafaxine will block only SERT. At increasing doses, NET will be inhibited; DAT will only be inhibited at higher desvenlafaxine doses.

The selective effects of desvenlafaxine on the anticholinergic, histaminergic and α adrenergic receptors are summarized as follows:

- ✓ **Anticholinergic Ach muscarinic affinity: Low. desv**enlafaxine has a low incidence of side effects of dry mouth, constipation, blurred vision and drowsiness.

- ✓ **Histaminergic H1 affinity**: Low. **Desv**enlafaxine has a low incidence of side effects of sedation and weight gain.

- ✓ **α 1 adrenergic affinity**: Low. **Desv**enlafaxine has a low incidence of side effects of hypotension, dizziness, drowsiness and other cardiovascular effects

Pharmacokinetics of desvenlafaxine

Desvenlafaxine has **linear pharmacokinetics,** and it does not inhibit its own metabolism. Each dose increase of desvenlafaxine may lead to a proportionately greater increase in the desvenlafaxine plasma levels.

Desvenlafaxine has Cmax of 260ng/ml. In comparison, the venlafaxine XR formulation resulted in a lower Cmax 150ng/ml while the venlafaxine IR formulation (Cmax 225ng/ml). In addition, desvenlafaxine Cmax increased by 16% when it is taken with food. However, the increased of Cmax by the presence of food did not show any clinical significance, thus desvelfaxine can be taken without regard to meals.

Time to peak plasma levels (Tmax.): 9 hours (

Steady state: Desvenlafaxine will reach plasma steady state within **4-5 days** of daily use.

Absorption: Desvenlafaxine is well absorbed by the

gastrointestinal system..

Bioavailability 80%

Protein binding: 30%. Desvenlafaxine has low protein binding properties and it is independent of drug concentration.

Half-Life: (t1/2): 10 hours

Metabolism: Desvenlafaxine is primarily metabolized by the liver via the enzyme CYP450: **3A4** into an inactive metabolite. It appears that desvenlafaxine metabolism is not affected by cytochrome 2D6.

Elimination: Urine. 45% of desvenlafaxine is excreted unchanged in urine at 72 hours after oral administration

P-gp system

Desvenlafaxine does not inhibit the P-gp transporter and is not expected to affect the pharmacokinetics of drugs that are substrate of the P-gp transporter.

How supplied

Desvenlafaxine 50mg, 100mg.

Dose range

- For depression: 50 mg – 100 mg

How to treat

- **For depression:** start desvenlafaxine with a maximal daily dose of 50mg once daily, to be increased, if no response to a maximum of 100mg once daily.

When and how to take the medication

Desvenlafaxine should be taken preferably in the morning as a once daily dose. The patient must avoid crushing or chewing the capsule as it will interfere with the drug absorption.

Clinical indications of Desvenlafaxine

- Major depression

Major Depressive Disorder (MDD)

Desvenlafaxine has established its efficacy in the treatment of MDD against placebo at dosesages ranging from 50mg/day to 400mg/day. Other study of desvelafaxine against the SSRI escitalopram at doses of 10mg-20mg/day showed comparable efficacy. Likewise similar results of equal efficacy were shown in another comparative study of desvenlafaxine to venlafaxine XR. Desvenlafaxine at doses of 200mg/day and 400mg/day were superior to placebo (14). However, only the 200mg/day of desvenlafaxine dose showed better remission rates than those of placebo.

Potential advantages for the use of desvenlafaxine

- Desvenlafaxine (the active metabolites of venlafaxine), has a *low affinity for the CYP 2D6 isoenzymes*, which may result in a lower risk of drug interactions.
- Desvenlafaxine has a low *affinity* for the α-adrenergic, histaminergic and the muscarinic receptors, thereby reducing the unwanted side effects of venlafaxine. This may result in better adherence to treatment.

How to stop the use of Desvenlafaxine

Due to its relatively short half-life, there is a need for a slow tapering of desvenlafaxine in order to avoid withdrawal symptoms.

Clinical implication: desvenlafaxine requires a gradual dose reduction in order to avoid the discontinuation symptoms. The desvenlafaxine dose should be given as a full dose of 50mg but not every day. In the event of getting withdrawal symptoms re instate of the previous dose of 50mg, and once the discontinuation symptoms disappear, desvenlafaxine should be taper off slowly over a longer period of time. Discontinuation symptoms have been reported when switching patients from venlafaxine to desvenlafaxine. Tapering of the initial antidepressant may be required to reduce discontinuation symptoms.

How long it takes to get an antidepressant effect

In order to get an antidepressant effect, desvenlafaxine should be used daily for at least 2 – 4 weeks. Like all antidepressants desvenlafaxine needs time before a substantial mood improvement emerges.

Side effects of desvenlafaxine

Desvenlafaxine's side effects are probably related to its ability to increase serotonin and norepinephrine levels in the brain.

Most side effects of desvenlafaxine develop soon after the initiation of treatment, and are dose-dependent, meaning the higher the dose of desvenlafaxine, the more prominent the side effects become. In most cases, desvenlafaxine side effects will gradually subside over time. The most common side effects of desvenlafaxine are nausea, dizziness, insomnia, anxiety, decreased appetite, constipation and sweating.

The nervous system

- Insomnia
- Nervousness

- Anxiety
- Dizziness
- Somnolence
- Tremor
- Disturbance in attention
- Abnormal dreams
- Jittery
- Chills
- Fatigue
- Vertigo
- Tinnitus
- Hot flushes
- Yawning
- Syncope
- Convulsion
- Dystonia
- Bruxism
- Musculoskeletal stiffness
- asthenia

Cardiac

No clinical differences were observed between desvenlafaxine treated patients and placebo treated patients for QT, PR and QRS.

Patients getting desvenlafaxine should have a regular monitoring of their blood pressure since increases in BP were observed.

Gastro intestinal

- Decreased appetite
- Nausea
- Dry mouth
- Vomiting
- Constipation

- Urinary retention
- Rash
- Photosensitivity
- alopecia

Sexual

- Decreased sex drive
- Delayed ejaculation
- Ejaculation failure
- Impotence
- Anorgasmia

Suicide

The FDA requires all antidepressants to carry a black box warning stating that antidepressants may increase the risk of suicide in persons under the age of 25 years. This warning is based on data suggesting that suicidal ideations and behavior has a 2-fold increase in children and in adolescents, and a 1.5 – fold increase in the 18 – 24 age group.

Desvenlafaxine side effects that need immediate attention

- Confusion
- Excitation
- Onset of seizure
- Yellow skin / eyes
- Severe allergic reaction
- Irregular heart beat
- Hypertension
- Induction of manic or hypomanic episode
- Activation of suicidal ideation and behaviour

Desvenlafaxine discontinuation reaction

The sudden discontinuation of venlafaxine can be associated with a discontinuation reaction, which is self-limiting. The most common symptoms of desvenlafaxine discontinuation reaction are:

- Irritability
- Agitation
- Dizziness
- Nausea
- Diarrhea
- sweating

A gradual down-titration of desvenlafaxine often reduces the risk of developing a discontinuation reaction.

Safety profile of desvenlafaxine

Use in pregnancy: Risk category C

There is a limited information regarding desvenlafaxine use in pregnant women.

Studies with desvenlafaxine in rats and rabbits showed no evidence of teratogenicity at doses up to 30 times the human dose of 100mg/day. Furthermore wehen desvelfaxine was administered to pregnant rats and rabbits during the period of organogenesis at doses up to 300mg/day, no teratogenic effects were observed.

However, the use of desvenlafaxine during the first trimester as well as throughout the pregnancy is not recommended.

Use during lactation

Desvenlafaxine is secreted in the breast milk.

Due to its unknown effects on the newborn's normal growth and development, breast feeding should be avoided in women who are using desvenlafaxine.

Special considerations with the use of desvenlafaxine

- **Narrow-angle glaucoma**: Desvenlafaxine may increase eye pressure due to its ability to potentiate the effects of norepinephrine (NE). Desvenlafaxine should be avoided in patients having un-controlled narrow-angle glaucoma as it may trigger an angle closure attack in patients with anatomically narrow angles.
- **Hypertension**: The Desvenlafaxine potentiating effects on norepinephrine (NE) can lead to increased heart rates and blood pressure.
- **Abnormal bleeding**: Desvenlafaxine may lead to abnormal bleeding and bruising. Concomitant use of warfarin, NSAIDs and aspirin may add to this risk.
- **Urinary hesitancy**: Desvenlafaxine's ability to potentiate norepinephrine (NE) can increase urethral resistance, which might lead to urinary hesitancy.
- **Alcohol**. Althought clinical studies has shown that desvenlafaxine does not increase the motor skills and cognitive impairment caused by alcohol, nevertheless, patients should be advised to avoid alcohol consumption while taking desvenlafaxine.

Desvenlafaxine drug interactions

Follows a list of desvenlafaxine's drug interactions

- **MAOI:** The concomitant use may cause CNS toxicity serotonin syndrome. Wait 21 days after the MAOI was stopped before initiating treatment with desvenlafaxine. After discontinuing

desvenlafaxine, wait 7 days before starting a MAOI.
- **Serotonergic drugs:** The concomitant use may increase the potential for serotonin syndrome.
- **NSAID**: The concomitant use may potentiate the risk of bleeding.
- **Warfarin**: potential pharmacologic interaction with increased risk of bleeding.
- **Triptans**: Potential interaction which may cause serotonin syndrome.
- **Lithium**: Potential interaction which may cause serotonin syndrome.
- **Venlafaxine:** Do not use both concomitantly.
- **St. John's Wort:** Potential interaction which may cause serotonin syndrome.

Warnings for desvenlafaxine

Pregnancy: Risk category C. Try to avoid use during pregnancy or breastfeeding. Assessment of the risks versus benefits must be discussed with the patient.

- **Suicide in children & young adults**: Desvenlafaxine may cause an increase in suicidal risk in young adults, and it carries a black box warning.
- **Serotonin syndrome**: Desvenlafaxine may cause serotonin syndrome. Serotonin syndrome symptoms include agitation, dizziness, hallucinations, delirium, seizures and coma along with autonomic instability, which includes tachycardia, fluctuating blood pressure, flushing, hyperthermia, tremor, muscular rigidity, myoclonus, hyperreflexia, and incoordination. The concomitant use of desvenlafaxine with a MAOI may precipitate serotonin syndrome which may be fatal.

- **MAOI**: Desvenlafaxine requires a *1 week washout period* before starting treatment with a MAOI. After a MAOI is stopped a *3- week washout period* is required before starting desvenlafaxine.
- **Renal impairment**: Desvenlafaxine requires a lower dose in mild to moderate renal impairment. In renal impaired patients, desvenlafaxine should be given in alternate days only.
- **Liver insufficiency**: Desvenlafaxine should be given at a maximum dose of 50mg/day in patients with moderate to severe hepatic impairment.
- **Mania & hypomania**: Desvenlafaxine, like all other antidepressants, may trigger mania in predisposed patients. The incidence of mania during the use of desvenlafaxine was **0.02%** Desvenlafaxine should be used cautiously in patients with a history of bipolar mood disorder.
- **Elderly**: Desvenlafaxine should be given at the lower dose of 50mg/day when it is used in the elderly.
- **Seizure**: Cases of seizure have been reported with desvenlafaxine. Desvenlafaxine should be used with caution in patients with seizure disorder.
- **Hyponatremia**: Hyponatremia may occur as the result of treatment with desvenlafaxine. Symptoms of hyponatremia include headache, poor concentration, confusion, memory impairment, weakness, unsteadiness and falls should be monitored. Severe acute symptoms of hyponatremia may include syncope, hallucination, seizure, coma and respiratory arrest.

Overdose with desvenlafaxine

There is limited clinical information with desvenlafaxine overdosage in human. No fatalities have been reported when desvenlafaxine was taken as monotherapy.

However overdose information with the parent drug venlafaxine showed that it can be lethal. Data from the U.K suggests that venlafaxine overdose carries a higher rate of lethality when compared with SSRI overdose. Death was reported following ingestion of very large doses of venlafaxine. Venlafaxine plasma levels within the range of 10 -90 mg/L was associated with fatalities. In addition, the concomitant use of venlafaxine with alcohol and/ or with other central nervous depressants such as painkillers or benzo-diazepines may result in death caused by respiratory depression.

The most common symptoms of desvenlafaxine overdose are

- Tachycardia
- Somnolence
- Mydriasis
- Seizure
- Vomiting
- ECG changes (QT prolongation, BBB
- Bradycardia
- Hypotension
- Vertigo
- Liver necrosis
- Serotonin syndrome
- Rhabdomyolysis
- coma

What to do in the case of desvenlafaxine overdose

In general, there is no antidote for desvenlafaxine overdose. Management is mainly supportive, aimed at maintaining respiration, pulse and blood pressure. In the event of a recent overdose with desvenlafaxine, a stomach washout with activated charcoal might help in the elimination of the un-absorbed drug and is done with a large bore oro-gastric tube with appropriate airway protection. The aim of the stomach lavage is to get rid of the drug leftovers.

In some ER departments, ipecac is also used in order to induce vomiting of the ingested toxin, however **induction of emesis is not recommended in semi-comatose and comatose patients.**

Due to the large volume of distribution of desvenlafaxine, forced diuresis, dialysis hemo-perfusion and exchange transfusion are unlikely to be effective.

Keeping open the patient's airway is compulsory, especially in semi - comatose individuals. The patient should be placed on his side in order to prevent aspiration of the vomitus back to the lungs. Suffocation due to vomit is the leading cause of death in venlafaxine overdose. Blood pressure and heart rate monitoring is very important. Fluid intake should be monitored with intravenous infusion of saline, and urinary output should also be carefully monitored. In most cases, desvenlafaxine overdose, requires hospitalization of the patient for at least 24 hours for intense observation.

Venlafaxine references.

1. Nemeroff, CB, Willard, L. Et al: venlafaxine and SSRI: Pooled remission analysis. New research poster presented at the 156th APA annual meeting , San Francisco, CA, May2003; 17-22.

2 Schmitt A.B, Bauer, M. et al. Differential effects of venlafaxine in the treatment of MDD according to baseline severity. European Archives of Psychiatry and Clinical Neuroscience, 2009;259, 329 – 339.

3 Kornstein, S.G, Mao, .Y et al. Escitalopram versus SNRI antidepressants in the acute treatment of major depressive disorder. CNS Spectrums, 2009;14(6), 326-333.

4 Davidson J.R, Meoni P. et al,. Archieving remission with venlafaxine and fluoxetine in major depression: its relationship to anxiety symptoms. Depression and anxiety, 2002;16(1), 4-13.

5 Thase, M.E, Entsuah, et al. Relative antidepressant efficacy of venlafaxine and SSRIs: sex- age interaction. Journal of woman Health, 2005;14, 6009-616.

6 Papakostas G.I, Thase M.E, Fava M. et al. Are antidepressant drugs that combine serotonergic and noradrenergic mechanisms of action more effective than the selective serotonin reuptake inhibitors in treating MDD? A meta analysis of studies of newer agents. Biological Psychiatry 2007;62, 1217 – 1227.

7 Benkert,O., Grunder, G, Wetzel, H et al. A randomized double blind comparison of a rapid escalating dose of venlafaxine and imipramine in inpatients with MDD and melancholia. Journal of Psychiatric Research, 1996;30(6), 441 – 451.

8 Rickels K., Pollack M., Sheehan D. et al. Efficacy of XR venlafaxine in non – depressed outpatients with GAD. Am. J. Psychiatry 2000;157: 968 – 974.

9 Allgulander C, Hackett D, Salinas E et al. Venlafaxine ER in the treatment of GAD: twenty – four week placebo – controlled dose – ranging study. Br J. Psychiatry 2001;179:15-22.

10 Allgulander C., Mangano R, Zhang J, et al Efficacy of

venlafaxine ER in patients with SAD. A double blind, placebo - controlled , parallel group comparison with Paroxetine. Human Psychopharmacology 2004;19: 387 - 396.

11 Flanagan, R.J,. Fatal toxicity of drugs used in psychiatry. Human Psychopharmacology, 2008;23 (Supp. 1), 43 - 51.

12 Wilson A. D, Howell, C, & Waring, W. Venlafaxine ingestion is associated with rhabdomyolysis in adults: A case serie. J. of Toxicological Sciences, 2007;32 (1), 97 - 101.

13 Clerc GE, Ruimy P, Verdeau- Pailes J. A double blind comparison of venlafaxine and fluoxetine in patients hospitalized for MDD and melancholia. Int. Clin. Psychopharmacol. 1994; 9:139-143.

14 Septien- Velez L, Pitroski B., Padmanahan SK et al, . A randomized double blind, placebo controlled trial of desvenlafaxine succinate in the treatment of MDD. Int. Clin. Psychopharmacol. 2007;22:338-347.

15 Lieberman, D.Z, Montgomery, SA, Tourian, K et al. A pooled analysis of two placebo - controlled trials of desvenlafaxine in major depressive disorder. Int. Clin. Psychopharmacol.2008; 23 (4), 188 - 197.

10

Duloxetine

Brand name: Cymbalta, Cymgen, Yelate

Mode of action: Duloxetine

1. Duloxetine is a Serotonin Reuptake Transporter(*SERT*) antagonist. The SERT is located on the pre synaptic nerve cell and is responsible for the transport of the excess free serotonin available in the synapse, back to the presynaptic nerve cell. Therefore duloxetine leads to increased serotonin in the synapse.

2. Duloxetine is a Norepinephrine Reuptake Transporter (NET) antagonist: The NET, located on the pre-synaptic nerve cell, is responsible for pumping the excess of norepinephrine from the synapse back to the pre synaptic nerve cell. The inhibition of NET results in more norepinephrine to be present in the synapse. Duloxetine inhibition of the NET is stronger than that of the SERT.

3. Duloxetine is a Dopamine Reuptake Transporter *(DAT)* antagonist: The DAT, located on the pre synaptic nerve cell, is responsible for pumping the excess of dopamine (DA) from the synapse back to the pre synaptic nerve cell. The inhibition of the DAT results in more dopamine to be present in the synapse. It appears that the inhibitory effects of duloxetine on the DAT are much more prominent in the frontal cortex.

The inhibitory effects on the SERT, NET and DAT transporters is effective within all of the duloxetine dosing range. Thus, even on lower doses, duloxetine is capable of blocking the serotonin, the norepinephrine and the dopamine reuptake transporters.

The selective effects of duloxetine on the serotonin, anticholinergic, histaminergic and α adrenergic receptors are summerized as follows:

- ✓ **Serotonin receptors affinity: High** 5-HT1A, 5-HT1B, 5 –HT1D, 5-HT2A and 5-HT2C. It appears that the inhibition of these post synaptic 5-HT receptors contributes to duloxetine's anti- anxiety and mood elevating properties.

- ✓ **Muscarinic receptors affinity: Low.** The inhibition of the muscarinic receptors can cause constipation, dry mouth and blurred vision.

- ✓ **Histamine H1 receptor affinity: Low.** The inhibition of the histaminergic receptors can result in excessive drowsiness.

- ✓ **α1 adrenergic receptor affinity: Low.** The inhibition of the α1 adrenergic receptors may cause low blood pressure.

Overall, the inhibitory effects of duloxetine on the 5-HT post synaptic receptors as well as on the histamine H1, anticholinergic muscarinic and α1 adrenergic receptors are weak and result in a favourable side effect profile compared to that of the old tricyclics (TCA) medications.

Pharmacokinetics of Duloxetine

Duloxetine has **linear pharmacokinetics,** and it does not inhibit its own metabolism. Thus, any dose increase of duloxetine may lead to a higher proportionate change in the drug plasma levels. The higher the daily dose of duloxetine, the higher the plasma level will get.

Peak plasma levels (Tmax): 6 hours.

Steady State: Daily use will lead to a plasma steady state within 3 days. Furthermore, steady state is often associated with a significant reduction in the side effects.

Absorption: Duloxetine is well absorbed by the gastrointestinal system. There is a 2-3 hours lag until absorption begins (Tlag=3H). The presence of food in the stomach may prolong the time needed to reach peak plasma concentration to between 6 to 10 hours. Drugs that raise the gastric pH may cause an earlier release of duloxetine.

However, duloxetine's enteric coating starts to dissolve in acidic environment were pH exceeds 5.5. However, in extremely acidic environments duloxetine may undergo hydrolysis to form naphthol.

The co-administration of duloxetine with magnesium or aluminium-containing anta acids has limited effect on its absorption.

Protein bounding: 95%. Duloxetine is highly bound to protein, mainly albumin or to α1-acidglycoprotein. Due to this highly protein bound state, the coadministration of other drugs that are also highly protein bound may result in an increase of their free plasma concentration which may cause adverse reactions.

Bioavailability: is 50%. Is lowered by one third in smokers. In elderly females, duloxetine bioavailability may increase by 25%.

Volume of distribution: Duloxetine volume of distribution is 1640 L.

Duloxetine elimination half-life (t 1/2): 12 hours.

This allows once-daily dosing. The half-life of duloxetine is not affected by gender. However, due to its relative short half- life and the lack of therapeutic effect of its principal metabolite, abrupt cessation of duloxetine can cause discontinuation syndrome.

Metabolism: Duloxetine is primarily metabolized by the liver via the enzyme CYP450: **1A2 and 2D6.**

The principal plasma metabolites of duloxetine are the *4- hydroxy duloxetine glucuronide* and the *5- hydroxy, 6 - methyl duloxetine sulphate.*

Only traces of unchanged duloxetine (less than 1%) are found in the urine while the majority (70%) of duloxetine, is excreted in the urine in the metabolite form.

Patients treated with agents who are also metabolized by 1A2 and 2D6 isoenzymes require monitoring their plasma levels and probably will require lower doses, as the concomitantly- used medication may accumulate in the plasma due to the inhibition of their metabolism via the liver iso- enzymes.

Patients with liver disease can experience a significant decrease in duloxetine metabolism. The half-life of duloxetine in cirrhotic patients appears to be 3 times longer compared to patients with healthy uncompromised livers. Similarly, in patients with end-stage renal disease, the Cmax levels may increase by 100% after taking even one single dose of 60mg duloxetine as compared to patients with normal kidney function.

Therefore, duloxetine should be avoided in people with compromised livers, heavy alcohol abusers and in those patients with renal impairments.

P-gp System

Duloxetine may **inhibit** the functions of P-gp in vivo and in vitro (4). The inhibitory effects of duloxetine on the P-gp system may interfere with the plasma levels of co- administered drugs which are also P-gp substrates.

Elimination: Urine 70%, Faeces 20%. The elimination of duloxetine may be increased by one third if its taken at night compared to the morning. Thus it is recommended to take duloxetine in the morning.

How supplied

- Capsule 20mg, 30mg, 60 mg,

Dose range

- 30 mg – 60 mg for depression
- 60mg a day for diabetic peripheral neuropathic pain
- 60 mg for fibromyalgia
- 60 mg once a day for generalized anxiety disorder
- 40mg twice a day for stress urinary incontinence

Duloxetine clinical indications

- Major depression
- Generalised anxiety disorder
- Diabetic peripheral neuropathic pain
- Stress urinary incontinence
- Fibromyalgia
- Chronic muscular pain

Major Depressive Disorder (MDD)

Several studies have established the superiority of duloxetine over placebo in the treatment of major depression. Patients who were given duloxetine at doses of 60mg – 120mg showed a significant improvement in their depressive symptoms at all dose levels and were significantly better than those patients who were getting a placebo. The remission rates after 8 weeks of treatment with duloxetine were 50% as compared to 25% with the treatment of placebo (1).

The long term efficacy of duloxetine was clearly demonstrated in more than 30 studies that were able to prove the ability of duloxetine to prevent depressive relapse and recurrence, which are often associated with long-term treatment.

There is no evidence that duloxetine has a faster onset of action or better efficacy than other available antidepressants.

Figure 10.1 summarizes duloxetine's response and remission rates compared to paroxetine and placebo.

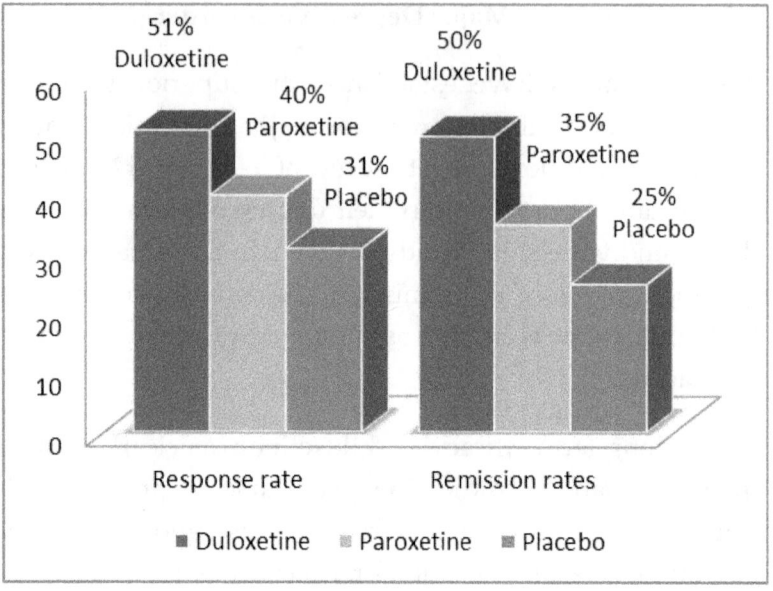

Figure 10.1: Comparison of the duloxetine response rates (Goldstein (2004) and the duloxetine remission rate (Thase 2007) versus paroxetine in the treatment of major depression. The response rate is defined as the % of patients having a 50% reduction in their HAM-D score between baseline and the end point.

Achieving remission is the main goal of all antidepressants as it favorably resonate on the patients mood and quality of life.

Stress induce urinary incontinence

Duloxetine's ability to reduce urine involuntary leakage associated with coughing, sneezing, bending or exercising was systematic reviewed (5).

The effects of duloxetine on urinary incontinence are probably related to its effects on serotonin and norepinephrine, both of which are involved in the regulation of the bladder and its sphincter function.

In some studies, duloxetine could reduce episodes of urinary incontinence by 50% at doses of 80mg a day(5). On the other hand, in a systematic review of non surgical treatments for urinary incontinence (6), duloxetine could improve urinary incontinence only in 11% of patients while pelvic floor muscle training combined with bladder training showed improvement in 36% of the cases.

Another clinical trial which compared duloxetine with pelvic floor muscle training (PFMT) showed mixed results (7). In this study 65% of patients who performed PFTM reported feeling better as compared to 54% of the patients on duloxetine.

However, the frequency of incontinence episodes decreased by 57% in the duloxetine group vs. 35% in the PFTM group. In this trial, 31% of the patients in the duloxetine group discontinued the trial due to the side effects.

Diabetic peripheral neuropathy

Duloxetine is approved for treatment of pain associated with diabetic peripheral neuropathy. Studies showed that 45% of the patients receiving duloxetine could achieve at least 50% reduction in pain as compared to only 20% of the placebo group patients.

The pain relief with duloxetine was achieved in the first two weeks of treatment at a dose of 60mg a day. Unfortunately duloxetine had only a minimal effect of the feeling of numbness and the tingling sensations, which are both commonly associated with diabetic neuropathic pain.

Generalised Anxiety Disorder (GAD)

Several double blind randomized controlled studies were able to show the effectiveness of duloxetine in the treatment of GAD at doses of 60mg a day (8).

Furthermore, it appears that long-term use with duloxetine may prevent GAD relapse.

Fibromyalgia

Duloxetine at doses of 60mg a day can reduce muscle pain and fatigue and improve the patient's reduced mental and physical functioning, regardless of the coexistence of depression. The favourable effects of duloxetine on fibromyalgia were more evident after one month of daily treatment with Duloxetine.

Muscle pain

Duloxetine was approved by the FDA for the treatment of chronic muscle pain, which includes low back pain and pain associated with osteoarthritis.

How to treat with duloxetine

- **For Major Depression (MDD)**: Start with 30 mg a day to be increased up to a maximum of 120mg a day.

- **For generalized anxiety disorder (GAD)**: Start with 30mg to be increased weekly up to a maximum of 120mg a day.

- **For fibromyalgia and neuropathic pain**: Start with 30 mg a day to be increased to a maximum of 60 mg a day. Doses above 60mg were associated with increased side effects.

When and how to take medication

Duloxetine should be taken preferably **in the morning** as a once a day dose, as evening use may result in its higher elimination rate.

Avoid crushing or chewing the capsule as it will interfere with the drug absorption. In the event of the patient having troubling side effects, the starting dose of 30 mg of duloxetine should continue for additional 3 – 7 days until the side effects subside, and only then consider a dose increase.

How to stop duloxetine

Due to its relative short half-life, there is a need for a slow tapering of duloxetine in order to avoid withdrawal symptoms.

In the event of the patient getting withdrawal symptoms reinstate the previous dose, and once the symptoms disappear, start reducing the duloxetine dose in a lower % and over longer period of time.

How long it takes to get an antidepressant effect

In order to get an antidepressant effect, duloxetine should be used daily for at least 2 – 4 weeks.

Although studies did not show increased efficacy above 60 mg a day, some patients might benefit from a higher dose up to 120 mg a day.

Side effects of duloxetine

Most side effects of duloxetine are probably related to its ability to increase serotonin and norepinephrine in the brain. The side effects of duloxetine develop soon after the initiation of treatment and often disappear with time. The most common side effects of duloxetine are:

Nervous system

- Insomnia

- Restlessness
- Restless leg syndrome
- Muscle spasm
- Tremor
- Hot flushes
- Headache
- Dizziness
- Seizures (rare and is mainly associated with upon treatment discontinuation)
- Increased sweating
- Fatigue
- Somnolence
- Rash

Psychiatric

- Lethargy
- Dyskinesia
- Myoclonus
- Poor sleep
- Increases stage 3 sleep
- Suppresses rapid eye movement (REM) sleep
- Paraesthesia
- Disturbed attention

Cardiac

- Palpitation
- Myocardial infraction
- Tachycardia

Gastro intestinal

GI symptoms are highly prominent with duloxetine use. The gastro intestinal side effects can develop within 30 minutes of drug ingestion, and they are more likely the result of the direct effect of duloxetine on the intestinal mucosa rather then the plasma peak level.

- Decreased appetite
- Nausea
- Vomiting
- Dry mouth
- Diarrhea
- Constipation
- Possible weight loss
- Gastritis

Sexual manifestations

The effects of duloxetine on sexual functioning are probably related to its effects on serotonin and are more prominent in males than in females.

- Decreased sex drive
- Delayed ejaculation
- Impotence
- Abnormal orgasm

Renal

- Dysuria
- Nocturia
- Polyuria
- Micturition urgency
- Abnormal urine odor

Musculoskeletal

- Musculoskeletal pain
- Muscle twitching

Eye manifestation

- Diplopia
- Visual disturbance
- Blurred vision

In general, duloxetine side effects are dose dependent: the higher the dose of duloxetine, the worse the side effect. Lowering the dose of duloxetine is often associated with the resolution of the side effects.

Post marketing reports of adverse reactions to duloxetine include anaphylactic shock, aggression, angioneurotic edema, erythema multiforme, Extrapyramidal disorder, glaucoma, gynecological bleeding, hallucinations, hypertensive crisis, muscle spasm, restless legs syndrome, trismus, urticarial and Stevens-johnson syndrome.

Suicide

The FDA requires all antidepressants to carry a black box warning stating that antidepressant may increase the risk of suicide in persons under the age of 25 years. This warning is based on data suggesting that suicidal ideations and behavior has a 2- fold increase in children and in adolescents, and a 1.5 - fold increase in the 18 - 24 age group.

Duloxetine side affects that requires immediate attention:

- Confusion
- Excitation
- Onset of seizure
- Yellow skin / eye
- Severe allergic reaction
- Irregular heart beats
- Hypertension

- Induction of manic or hypomanic episode
- Activation of suicidal ideation and behaviour

Physical & psychological dependence

In animal studies, duloxetine did not show abuse potential. Furthermore, in human clinical trials, there was no indication of drug-seeking behaviour. However, duloxetine produces physical dependence, as evidenced by the presence of withdrawal symptoms upon abrupt discontinuation of the drug. This physical dependence to duloxetine is similar to other SNRI and SSRI drugs. Clinicians should carefully monitor the patients for signs of misuse or abuse.

Duloxetine discontinuation reaction

A sudden discontinuation of duloxetine can be associated with a discontinuation reaction which is self-limiting. The most common symptoms of discontinuation reaction are:

- Irritability
- Agitation
- Dizziness
- Electric shock sensations
- Anxiety
- Confusion
- Headache
- Lethargy
- Insomnia
- Seizures
- Dysphoric mood

A slow down titration of duloxetine is often reduces the risk of having the discontinuation reaction.

Safety profile of duloxetine

Use in pregnancy: FDA rik category C

Duloxetine is not evidently teratogenic. In studies on pregnant rats with doses of duloxetine up to of 7 times of the maximum recommended human dose (MRHD), there was no evidence of teratogenicity.

The risk of pregnant mothers with a history of depression to develop depression during their pregnancy and especially after child delivery is very high and often requires the continuation of the treatment with SSRIs during and after the pregnancy.

However, the use of duloxetine during the first trimester as well as throughout the pregnancy is not recommended. Newborn children exposed to duloxetine in the maternal third trimester may develop respiratory distress, cyanosis, apnea vomiting, hypoglycemia, hypotonia, hypertonia, tremor, jitteriness, irritability and continues crying spells as well as feeding difficulties, temperature instability and seizures. These symptoms may result in prolonged hospitalization and respiratory support and tube feeding.

Use during lactation

Duloxetine is secreted in the breast milk of lactating woman. The estimated daily infant dose is approximately 0.14% of that of the maternal dose. The steady state concentration of duloxetine in the breast milk is 25% of the plasma concentration. Due to its unknown effects on the newborn's normal growth and development, breast feeding should be avoided.

Use of duloxetine in the pediatric population

Duloxetine is not approved for use in pediatric patients. The safety and effectiveness of duloxetine in the pediatric population have not been established.

However, duloxetine as all other antidepressant medications may increase the risk, compared to placebo, of suicidal thinking and behavior in children and young adult. Thus, the use of duloxetine in this population must balance the risk with the clinical need. Families and caregivers are advised to observe closely for clinical worsening, suicidality or unusual change in behaviour.

Duloxetine drug interaction

Duloxetine drug interactions aredue to its metabolism by the liver enzyme CYP 450: 2D6 and 1A2 .

Follows a list of duloxetine drug interactions with the possible clinical consequences.

- **Warfarin:** The concomitant use may displace warfarine from its protein. Increase INR may cause increased risk of of bleeding.
- **Fluvoxamine:** The concomitant use may result in 2.5-fold increase in duloxetine peak plasma concentration and 3 fold increase in duloxetine half- life. High plasma levels of duloxetine may increase the risk of hypertension, increased heart rates, syncope and a possible serotonin syndrome.
- **Smoking:** Smoking is associated with **30% decrease** in duloxetine plasma concentration.
- **MAOI;** The concomitant use may cause CNS toxicity - serotonin syndrome. Patient must wait 21 days after MAOI was stopped before initiating treatment with duloxetine and wait 7 days to start a MAOI after discontinuing duloxetine.
- **Zolpidem:** The concomitant use may cause delirium.
- **Beta blockers:** The concomitant use may increase duloxetine plasma levels.

- **Paroxetine, Quinidine & Fluoxetine:** The concomitant use may increase the concentration of duloxetine AUC by 60%.
- **Triptans, Lithium, Linezolid, Tramadol, St. John's Wort:** the concomitant use may result in serotonin syndrome.

Warnings for duloxetine

- **Pregnancy: Risk category C.** Try to avoid use during pregnancy or breastfeeding. Assessment of the risks versus benefits must be discussed with the patient.
- **Liver impairment:** Duloxetine is associated with a dose-dependent risk of liver enzyme elevation which can be evident after two month of treatment. There have been reports of fatal liver failure in patients treated with duloxetine. The clinical presentation consists of abdominal pain, jaundice, hepatomegaly, increased transaminase blood level to 20 times higher the upper normal limits. Duloxetine must be discontinuing in patient who develop jaundice.
- **Alcohol:** Due to the possible effects of duloxetine and alcohol on the liver, duloxetine must not be given to heavy alcohol users. Increase in liver transaminase less then 3 times the upper limit of normal ALT occurred only in 1.37% of treated patients with duloxetine.
- **Mydriasis:** Duloxetine is associated with an increased risk of mydriasis due to its ability to potentiate the effects of norepinephrine (NE). Duloxetine should be avoided in patients having uncontrolled narrow-angle glaucoma.
- **Syncope:** Duloxetine's potentiating effects on norepinephrine (NE) can lead to increased heart rates and blood pressure. However orthostatic hypotension and syncope have been reported with duloxetine mostly in the first week of treatment or after duloxetine dose increases.
- **ECG:** Duloxetine has no clinical effects on the ECG profile and on the QTc interval. It has been shown to be safe in

the treatment of depression in patients with history of myocardial infraction and angina.

- **Urinary hesitancy**: Duloxetine's ability to potentiate norepinephrine (NE) may increase urethral resistance which may cause urinary hesitancy.
- **Bleeding**: Duloxetine may increase the risk of bleeding especially whenever it is used with aspirin, warfarin and non steroidal anti-inflammatory (NSAIDs) drugs. In most cases, the bleeding is mild and episodic and consists of hematomas, epistaxis and petechiae. However, life-threatening haemorrhages can occur.
- **Serotonin syndrome** There have been reports of serotonin syndrome with the use of duloxetine alone and more frequently in combination with other serotoninergic drugs such as triptans, antipsychotics and other dopamine antagonists, and with MAOIs. The most common symptoms of serotonin syndrome include agitation, hallucination, delirium and coma as well as autonomic instability which include labile blood pressure, hyperthermia and tachycardia and neuromuscular symptoms which include hyperreflexia and incoordination. Gastro intestinal symptoms can also be frequently present with serotonin syndrome and include nausea, vomiting and diarrhea. The concomitant use of duloxetine with MAOI is contra indicated while the concomitant use of duloxetine with tryptophan and triptans is not recommended. Duloxetine must be discontinued immediately if serotonin syndrome is suspected and careful monitoring of vital signs and autonomic parameters as well as supportive treatment should be initiated.

- **Discontinuation symptoms** for duloxetine are relatively infrequent with a rate of 14% and were similar to those of

SSRIs. The discontinuation symptoms of duloxetine include nausea, diarrhea, vomiting, dizziness, headache, tiredness, irritability, agitation, anxiety electric shock sensation, confusion, emotional lability tinnitus insomnia and seizures. Although the discontinuation symptoms are transient and self-limiting, a gradual reduction of the duloxetine dose is strongly recommended.

- **Hypomanic activation** was reported only in **0.1%** of duloxetine treated patients.
- **Seizure** developed only in **0.03%** of patients treated with duloxetine. However, patient with a history of seizure disorder should be given duloxetine with care.
- **Hypertension:** Duloxetine treatment was associated with mean increase of 0.5mmHg in systolic blood pressure and 0.8mm Hg in diastolic blood pressure. Despite this minimal effect of duloxetine on blood pressure, blood pressure should still be measured prior to initiating treatment with duloxetine.
- **Diabetes**: Duloxetine may worsen glycemic control in diabetic patients. Duloxetine was associated with a small increase in mean fasting blood glucose by 12mg/dl while the HbA1c was increased by 0.5%.
- **Urinary hesitation and retention** may be associated with duloxetine use and in some cases hospitalization and catheterization is required.
- **Hyponatremia**: Duloxetine use was associated with cases of clinically significant hyponatremia, especially in elderly patients who may be at greater risk.

- **MAOI:** Duloxetine combined use with MAOI may be fatal. Duloxetine requires **7 days** washout period before starting with MAOI. Duloxetine requires **3 weeks** washout period after MAOI was stopped.

- **Alcohol:** Duloxetine is not recommended in patients abusing alcohol.
- **Thioridazine:** Duloxetine must be avoided in patients who are using Thioridazine.
- **Renal impairment**: Duloxetine **does not** require any dose adjustment in mild to moderate renal impairment.

Duloxetine overdose

Duloxetine is **relatively safe in mono-therapy overdose**. Although most fatalities occurred with mixed drug overdoses, there are rare incidence of fatalities with duloxetine mono therapy at doses as low as 1000mg.

General symptoms of duloxetine overdose

Initially, the patient might feel extremely tired and lethargic. The pulse will slow down, and the breathing frequency will also decrease. As the level of intoxication increases, the level of consciousness will decrease, and the patient will become unresponsive to external stimulations. The reflexes will disappear, and the breathing will get shallow. The patient's pulse and blood pressure will drop until cardiovascular system collapse.

In general, concomitant use of duloxetine with alcohol and with other central nervous depressants such as painkillers or benzodiazepines may result in death cause by respiratory depression.

Symptoms of duloxetine over dose are

- vomiting
- somnolence, over sedation
- agitation
- dilated pupils
- abnormal heart rhythm

- hypotension/ hypertension
- syncope
- tachycardia
- seizures
- coma

What to do in the case of duloxetine overdose

In general, there is no antidote for duloxetine overdose and the management is mainly supportive which is aimed to maintain respiration, pulse and blood pressure. In the event of a recent overdose with duloxetine, a stomach washout with activated charcoal might help in the elimination of the un- absorbed drug.

In some ER departments, ipecac is also used in order to induce vomiting of the ingested toxin, however **induction of emesis is not recommended in semi- comatose and comatose patients**. Due to the large volume of distribution of duloxetine, forced diuresis, dialysis hemoperfusion and exchange transfusion are unlikely to be effective. Keeping open the patient's airway is compulsory, especially in semi - comatose individuals.

The patient should be placed on his side in order to prevent respiration of the vomitus back to the lungs. Suffocation due to vomit is the leading cause of death in duloxetine overdose. Blood pressure and heart rate monitoring is very important. Fluid intake should be monitored with intravenous infusion of saline, and urinary output should also be carefully monitored. In most cases, duloxetine overdose, requires hospitalization for at least 24 hours for intense observation.

Duloxetine references

1 Thase M.E, Pritchett, Y.L, Ossana, M.J et al. Efficacy of duloxetine and SRI: comparisons as assessed by remission rates in patients with MDD. Journal of clinical Psychopharmacology, 2007;27(6), 672-676.

2 Goldstein DJ, Lu, Y, Derke MJ et al. Duloxetine in the treatment of depression: a doublr blind placebo – controlled comparison with paroxetine. J. Clin Psychopharmacol 2004 24 389 – 399.

3 Stahl SM, Megan M., Grady BA et al. SNRIs Their pharmacology, clinical efficacy and tolerability in comparison with other classes of antidepressants. CNS spectrum 2005;volume 10 number 9 732 – 747.

4 Zao R.,Cao J.,Peng W. In vitro and in vivo evaluation of the effects of duloxetine on P-gp function. Human Psychopharmacology Clinical And Experimental. 2010;Volume 25,issue 7-8, 553-559.

5 Mariapan P, Ballantyne Z., N'Dow JM. Cochrane database Syst Rev. 2005;(3): CD 004742.

6 Shamliyan TA, Kane RL, Wyman J. et al. Systematic review: randomized controlled trials of nonsurgical treatments for urinary incontinence in woman. Ann. Intern. Med. 2008;148 (6): 459 – 473.

7 Trial 2615A efficacy and safety of duloxetine compared with placebo, pelvic floor muscle training in subjects with moderate to severe stress urinary incontinence. www.clinicalstudyresults.org/drugdetails/viewfile.php?.

8 Allgulander, C, Hartford, J, Russell, J. et al. Pharmacotherapy of GAD. Results of duloxetine treatment from pooled of three clinical

trials. Urrent Medical and research opinion, 2007;23(6), 1245 – 1252.

11

Fluoxetine

Brand name: Prozac

Mode of action

1. **Fluoxetine is a Serotonin Reuptake Transporter (SERT) antagonist.** The inhibition of the SERT, which is located on the presynaptic neurons, results in increased serotonin synaptic levels. Among the SSRIs, fluoxetine is the weakest inhibitor of SERT. In vivo, 20mg of fluoxetine is capable of occupying 76%-85% of SERTs, suggesting that the starting dose of fluoxetine is adequate to produce its clinical antidepressant effects.

2. **Fluoxetine is a 5-HT2C receptor antagonist:** The 5-HT2C receptors are located on the post synaptic nerve cell. The inhibition of the 5-HT2C receptors regulates the release of cortical dopamine and cortical norepinephrine, resulting in improved concentration, improved attention, increased energy levels and an overall activation effect, which is often seen at the early stages of treatment with fluoxetine.

3. **Fluoxetine desensitizes the 5-HT1A auto-receptor.** In normal conditions, the activation of the 5-HT1A somato dendrite pre-synaptic auto receptor will *turn off* the release of serotonin from the pre-synaptic nerve cell. Thus, desensitization of the 5-HT1A somato dendritic presynaptic auto receptors results in a substantial increase of serotonin release by the pre synaptic nerve cell.

The selective effects of fluoxetine on the anticholinergic, histaminergic and α adrenergic receptors are summarized as follows:

- ✓ **Anticholinergic Ach muscarinic affinity: Low.** Fluoxetine has low side effects of dry mouth, constipation, blurred vision and drowsiness.

- ✓ **Histaminergic H1 affinity**: **Low.** Fluoxetine has low side effects of sedation and weight gain.

- ✓ **α 1 adrenergic affinity**: **Low.** Fluoxetine has low side effects of hypotension, dizziness, drowsiness and other cardiovascular effects.

Pharmacokinetics of fluoxetine

Fluoxetine has a **Non-linear pharmacokinetics**. Fluoxetine has been shown to decrease its own metabolism by the inhibition of the liver enzymes cytochrome P450 2D6 which is the main enzyme responsible for fluoxetine metabolism. However, high daily doses of fluoxetine results in a significant reduction of 2D6 activity due to fluoxetine's ability to inhibit its own metabolism, which will cause higher blood levels of fluoxetine, and dose dependent side effects.

Thus, patients who had no side effects with fluoxetine at the beginning of treatment may experience newly emerged unwanted symptoms later on as the treatment continues.

Furthermore, any dose increase in fluoxetine may cause a disproportionate increase in the fluoxetine plasma levels which may cause serotonin-related side effects that consist of headache, vomiting, nausea, and abdominal discomfort.

In addition, the concomitant use of other psychoactive drugs which are also metabolized by the 2D6 liver enzymes may compete with fluoxetine, resulting in additional increases in fluoxetine blood levels.

Therefore, the concomitant use together with fluoxetine of beta blockers, risperidone, codeine, haloperidol, class 1C antiarrhythmics, tricyclics, venlafaxine, paroxetine, and bupropion, may result in increases in the blood levels of the concomitant medications as well as more adverse reactions.

Peak plasma levels *(tmax)*: **6 – 8 hours.**

Side effects of fluoxetine are dosed related and tend to emerge when the drug reaches its peak plasma level. A single dose of fluoxetine will reach its peak plasma level after 6-8 hours, resulting in emergence of serotonin related side effects.

Steady state: Regular use of fluoxetine results in steady plasma levels after four weeks of regular treatment, which is associated with a significant reduction in the side effects.

Absorption: Fluoxetine is rapidly absorbed through the intestine, and it is not altered by the presence or absence of food in the stomach. Although food may delay its absorption by 1-2 hours, it does not have any clinical implication. Thus fluoxetine can be taken with or without meals.

Bioavailability: 72%

Protein binding: 94.5% . Fluoxetine is highly protein bound to albumin and to α1 glycoprotein.

In addition, due to its elevated lipid solubility, and it's small molecular size, fluoxetine can readily pass through the blood – brain barrier in a very high proportion.

Fluoxetine's concentration in the brain drastically increases in the first five weeks of treatment. However, when the treatment with fluoxetine is stopped, there is a slow elimination of fluoxetine from the brain resulting in 50% decrease in fluoxetine brain levels after the first week of treatment discontinuation.

Measurement in the blood: The normal blood fluoxetine concentration is in the range of 50 – 500 µg/l. However, the quantification of fluoxetine blood levels has no clinical relevance and is only used for forensic purposes to confirm a diagnosis of poisoning or in the case of death investigations.

Half-life (t1/2): Fluoxetine 2-4 days;

 Norfluoxetine 7 – 15 days

Fluoxetine has an exceptionally **long half-life** as compared to all the other SSRIs. This long half- life of fluoxetine results in very long time needed for its elimination from the body, which may increase the risk of drug interactions long after fluoxetine was stopped. The drug interaction may cause undesired side effects, consisting of   headache, vomiting, nausea and abdominal discomfort.

On the other hand, the long half-life of fluoxetine results in a substantial reduced incidence of discontinuation reactions. Thus, fluoxetine can be added to paroxetine, which is another SSRI, in order to reduce the risk of paroxetine discontinuation side effects. Fluoxetine is a racemic mixture (50/50) of R- fluoxetine and S-fluoxetine enantiomers with equivalent pharmacological activity, although the S-enantiomer is eliminated more slowly and is the predominant enantiomer present in the plasma during the steady state.

Metabolism: Fluoxetine is primarily metabolized in the liver by the cytochrome P450 enzyme **2D6 to norfluoxetine**. About 7% of the population has reduced activity of the iso enzyme 2D6 resulting in poor metabolism of fluoxetine, TCAs, debrisoquin and dextromethorphan. Patients with a compromised liver such as in the case of liver cirrhosis or in the elderly, have reduced 2D6 efficiency and requires a lower dose of fluoxetine to avoid excessive accumulation of the drug. In patients with liver cirrhosis, the elimination half-life of fluoxetine was 8 days as compared to 2-4 days of healthy subjects.

Fluoxetine's principal metabolite, *norfluoxetine*, is three times more selective for SERT than the parent drug. In addition, after several weeks of fluoxetine intake, the plasma level of norfluoxetine is three times higher than that of fluoxetine.

The P-gp System

Fluoxetine is **an intermediate inhibitor of the P-gp** functions in vivo and in vitro (2). The inhibitory effects of fluoxetine on the P-gp system may interfere with the plasma levels of other co-administered drugs, which are also P-gp substrates. Furthermore, the P-gp system's presence in the blood brain barrier (BBB) may be an important factor limiting the brain entry of paroxetine as well as that of amitriptyline, venlafaxine, doxepine, citalopram and trimipramine (3).

Elimination: Urine 80% and Faeces 20%.

How supplied

- Tablet 10 mg,
- Capsules 10mg, 20 mg, 40 mg
- Liquid 20mg/5ml bottles and 120 ml bottles

Dose range

- 20 mg – 80 mg for depression
- Doses of 60 – 80 mg a day may be required for OCD and Bulimia.

Fluoxetine clinical indications

- Major depression
- Panic disorder
- Obsessive compulsive disorder

- Premenstrual dysphoric syndrome
- Bulimia

Major Depressive Disorder (MDD)

Several studies have established the superiority of fluoxetine over placebo in the treatment of depression. Fluoxetine treated patients showed a significant improvement in their depressive symptoms as early as the second week of treatment. However, within the SSRI class, there is no evidence for superior effectiveness of one agent over another. In addition, there is no direct relationship between fluoxetine plasma concentration and the clinical response. The efficacy of fluoxetine in MDD is illustrated in Figure 11.1.

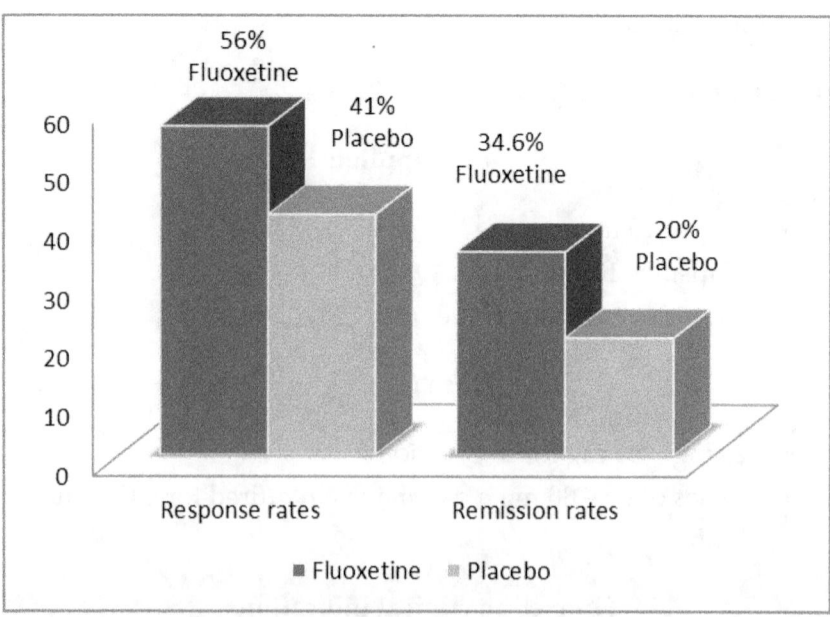

Figure 11.1 *1*. Fluoxetine response study. Adapted from Emslie G.J., Heiligenstein J., Wagner K.D , et al. Fluoxetine for acute treatment of depression in children and adolescent. J. of the

American academy of child and adolescent psychiatry. 2002;41, 1205-1215. **2 Fluoxetine remission study**. Adapted from Becch P., Cialdella P, Haungh M, et al. Meta analysis of randomized controlled trials of fluoxetine versus placebo and TCA in the short term of MDD. J. of Psychiatry. 2000;176: 421-428.

In addition, the efficacy of fluoxetine in relapse prevention was also extensively investigated. In a study conducted with 570 patients diagnosed with MDD (5), the patients were randomized into 12-week treatment with fluoxetine.

The 292 responders were randomly assigned to one of three arms: fluoxetine, with a mean dose of 45.8mg/day, or to fluoxetine mean dose of 8mg/day, or to placebo, for additional 52 weeks or until the patients relapsed.

After 52 weeks of treatment 45% of the fluoxetine treated patients relapsed as compared to 72% of the placebo-treated patients.

Those results clearly demonstrated the efficacy of fluoxetine in relapse prevention as illustrated in Figure 11.2

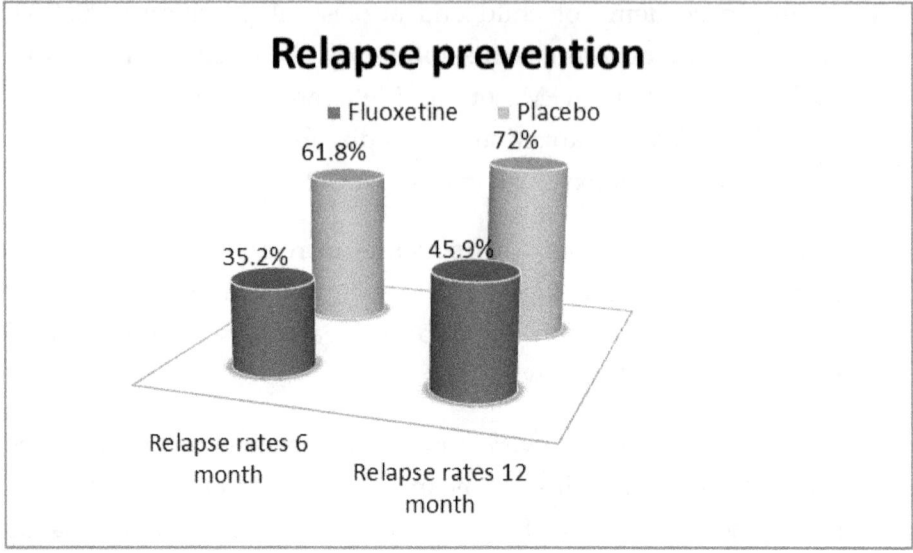

Figure 11.2: **Fluoxetine V Placebo relapse prevention study.** Adapted from Mcgareth PJ, Stewart J, Quitkin F, et al. Predictors of relapse in a prospective study of fluoxetine treatment of MDD. Am. J. Psychiatry 2006;163: 1542-1548 *(5)*

OCD

Fluoxetine has been shown to be effective in the treatment of OCD, independent of the patient's mood. Patients with OCD may require higher doses of fluoxetine ranging from 60-80 mg a day. The treatment with fluoxetine in OCD requires treatment for a longer period.

Bulimia

In general, any agent with the ability to block the SERT showed efficacy in the treatment of bulimia.

Studies with fluoxetine given in a dose range of 20- 60 mg a day, was shown to be efficacious on the frequency of binge eating, on increasing carbohydrate craving and on decreasing the purging behavior.

Premenstrual Dysphoric Disorder (PMDD)

Several studies showed that fluoxetine is effective in the treatment of PMDD. The recommended dose range of fluoxetine for PMDD is 20–60 mg a day.

Panic disorder (PD)

All SSRIs are highly effective for the treatment of PD. Due to the possible activation early in the treatment with fluoxetine, which may worsen the on-going panic attacks, the initial dose of fluoxetine should be 10 mg a day and it can be increased slowly up to 20 – 80 mg a day depending on the clinical results. Figure 9.4 illustrates a fluoxetine study in Panic disorder which resulted in 82% response rates to fluoxetine and only 42% remission rates after 6 weeks of treatment.

The efficacy of fluoxetine in PD is illustrated in Figure 11.3

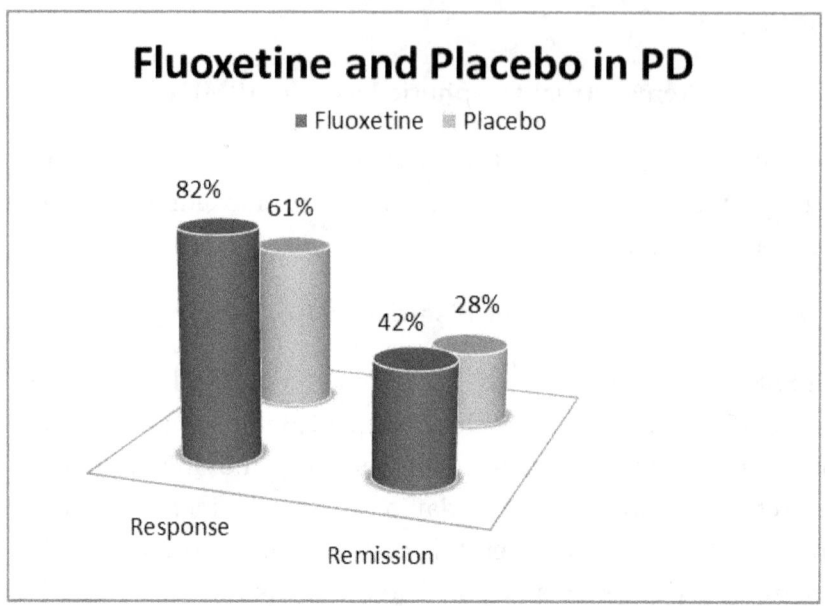

Figure 11.3 Fluoxetine versus placebo study in PD response & remission rates. Adapted from Michelson D, Allgolacher C, Danlofer K et al. Efficacy of usual antidepressant regims of fluoxetine in panic disorder. B. J. of psychiatry 2001;179: 514-518 (6).

How to treat with fluoxetine

Start with 20mg a day in a single morning dose. Activation-related symptoms may develop at the beginning of the treatment with fluoxetine, and consists of elevated energy, increased anxiety and irritability. In the event of activation, a lower dose of fluoxetine (10 mg) should be given at the initiation of treatment, and should be slowly increased up to 20mg a day.

How long it takes to get an antidepressant effect

In order to get an antidepressant effect, fluoxetine should be used daily for at least 2- 4 weeks. In some cases, dose increases may result in a better clinical response.

Like all antidepressants, fluoxetine requires time before a substantial mood improvement can be evident.

Fluoxetine side effects

Most side effects of fluoxetine are related to the increased levels of serotonin in the brain. Often, the side effects develop soon after the initiation of treatment with fluoxetine and disappear with time. The most common side effects of fluoxetine are:

Nervous system

- Insomnia
- Agitation, restlessness, jitteriness
- Akathisia
- Tremor, worsening motor symptoms of Parkinson's disease
- Increased sweating
- Flushing
- Headache
- Dizziness
- Seizures
- Mental slowing
- Reduced attention
- Apathy
- Emotional blunting
- Rash

Gastro intestinal

The gastro intestinal side effects can develop within 30 minutes of drug ingestion and are more likely the result of the direct effect of fluoxetine on the intestinal mucosa rather than of its plasma peak levels.

- Decreased appetite
- Nausea,
- vomiting
- dry mouth
- Diarrhea
- constipation
- Possible weight loss

Sexual

- Decreased sex drive
- Delayed ejaculation
- Impotence
- Inability to reach an orgasm

Suicide

The FDA requires all antidepressants to carry a black box warning stating that antidepressant may increase the risk for suicide in persons under the age of 25 years. This warning is based on data suggesting that suicidal ideations and behavior has a 2 fold increase in children and in adolescents, and a 1.5 – fold increase in the 18 – 24 age group.

Side effects that requires immediate attention: Stop the treatment with fluoxetine immediately.

- Confusion
- Excitation
- Onset of seizure

- Yellow skin / eyes
- Severe allergic reaction
- Irregular heart beats

Physical and psychological dependence

In animal studies, fluoxetine did not show abuse potential. Furthermore, in human clinical trials, there was no indication of drug seeking behaviour, euphoria and drug liking. However, fluoxetine can cause physical dependence, as evidenced by the presence of withdrawal symptoms upon abrupt discontinuation of the drug. This physical dependence on fluoxetine is similar to the other SNRIs and SSRIs.

In general, clinicians should carefully monitor the patients for signs of misuse or abuse

Safety profile of fluoxetine

Use in pregnancy: Risk level C

Fluoxetine **is not evidently teratogenic**. According to the FDA classification, fluoxetine is classified as having a **risk level C**.

The risk of pregnant mothers with a history of depression to develop depression during their pregnancy and especially after child delivery is very high and often requires the continuation of the treatment with SSRIs during and after the pregnancy.

The administration of fluoxetine to pregnant rats at doses 1.2 times the maximum recommended human dose (MRHD) produced no evidence of carcinogenicity.

Similarly, there was no evidence of genotoxic effects of fluoxetine on bacterial mutation assays or on mouse lymphoma assays.

Although the use of fluoxetine during the first trimester was not associated with higher rates of major malformations, yet there was a slightly higher rate of miscarriages as compared to woman treated with non- teratogenic medications.

Babies exposed to fluoxetine during late pregnancies had a higher risk of developing serotonergic toxicity. Newborn children exposed to fluoxetine in the maternal third trimester may develop respiratory distress, cyanosis, apnea vomiting, hypoglycemia, hypotonia, hypertonia, tremor, jitteriness, irritability and continuouess crying spells as well as feeding difficulties, temperature instability and seizures.

These symptoms may result in prolonged hospitalization and respiratory support and tube feeding.

As a result of such dangers, the FDA issued a warning for all SSRI to carry a risk for neonatal toxicity, and therefore, should not be taken by the mother before delivery.

Use during lactation

Fluoxetine is secreted in the breast milk. Due to its unknown effects on the new born's normal growth and development, breast feeding should be avoided. Assessing the risk versus benefits must be discussed with the patient.

Fluoxetine drug interaction

Follows a list of fluoxetine drug interaction:

- **Warfarin**: The concomitant use may cause Possible enhancement of warfarines anticoagulant effects thus leading to poor control of desired blood coagulation.
- **Carbamazepine:** The concomitant use may results in increased plasma levels of carbamazepine, phenytoin and valproate (up to 50%).

- **MAOI;** The concomitant use may cause CNS toxicity - serotonin syndrome. Patients must wait 5 weeks when switching from or to MAOIs.
- **Benzodiazepines:** The concomitant use may Increased plasma levels of alprazolam, diazepam and bromazepam.
- **Lithium:** The concomitant use may cause serotonin syndrome.
- **Clozapine & Haloperidol:** The concomitant use may Increased plasma levels of both antipsychotics medications.
- **Pindolol & Propranolol:** The concomitant use may Increased blood levels of beta-blockers which results in higher rates of lethargy and bradycardia. Moreover, can increase the half-life of Pindolol by 28%.
- **LSD:** The concomitant use may cause grand mal seizure.
- **Narcotics:** The concomitant use may D*ecreased the analgesic effects* of morphines, oxymorphone and hydromorphone. Concomitant use of fluoxetine with Tramadol can increase the risk of convulsions. Concomitant use of fluoxetine and pentazocine can lead to excitatory toxicity.
- **Protease inhibitors:** The concomitant use may **cause** Serotonin syndrome.
- **Sildenafile:** The concomitant use may cause Hypotension due to the inhibition of sildenafil metabolism.
- **Sumatriptans:** The concomitant use may cause serotonin syndrome.
- **Imipramine & Desipramine:** The concomitant use may cause Up to 10-fold increases in their plasma levels.

Precautions & special considerations

> **Pregnancy: Risk category C.** Try to avoid use during pregnancy or breastfeeding. Assessment of the risks versus benefits must be discussed with the patient.

- **Abnormal bleeding** may develop subsequent to the use of fluoxetine together with aspirin, warfarin and NSAIDs. Patients should be cautioned about the risk of bleeding associated with the concomitant use of fluoxetine with other drugs that affect coagulation.
- **Activation of hypomania or mania** occurred only in 0.1% of fluoxetine treated bipolar patients. However, it is generally believed that treatment with antidepressants may increase the likelihood of precipitation of a mixed manic episode in bipolar patients, requirings careful symptom monitoring, and detailed psychiatric history taking including family history of BMD, depression and suicide.
- **The incidence of seizures** occurred only in **0.1%** of fluoxetine treated patients. The low percentage of seizures appears to be equal to that associated with other antidepressant medications. However, fluoxetine should be given with care in patients with a history of seizures.
- **Discontinuation response** may develop upon sudden fluoxetine discontinuation. The most common discontinuation symptoms include dysphoric mood, agitation, anxiety, dizziness irritability, paresthesias in the form of electric shock sensations, headaches, insomnia, emotional lability, lethargy and confusion. Due to its long half-life, there is less need for a slow tapering of fluoxetine in order to avoid withdrawal symptoms. However, gradual dose reduction is strongly recommended.
- **Hyponatremia** may develop subsequent to the use of fluoxetine, especially in volume depleted patients and in patients on diuretics. It is possible that hyponatremia results from the syndrome of inappropriate antidiuretic hormone secretion (SIADH). The symptoms of hyponatremia include headaches, reduced concentration, confusion, weakness and unsteadiness, which may lead to

falls. Severe cases of hyponatremia may result in seizures, hallucinations, respiratory arrest, coma and death. Elderly patients appeared to be at a higher risk. The withdrawal of fluoxetine often results in symptom resolution.
- **Angle-closure glaucoma**: Fluoxetine may have an effect on the pupil size resulting in mydriasis. Patients with narrow angle glaucoma may experience increased intraocular pressure when treated with fluoxetine.
- **Weight loss & altered appetite**: Fluoxetine was associated with anorexia in 11% of treated patients, while 1.4% of the patients reported weight loss.
- **Suicide risk**: Fluoxetine may cause an increase in suicidal risk in young adults. Pooled analysis of trials of drugs used for MDD showed that SNRIs and SSRIs may increase the risk of suicidal thinking and behaviour in children, adolescents and young adults aged 18-24. The use of antidepressants in this population must balance the risk of suicide with the clinical need. Careful monitoring of the patient's clinical worsening, and suicidality should also involve the family and all other caregivers.
- **MAOI**: Fluoxetine requires a 5 weeks washout before starting with MAOI as the concomitant use of fluoxetine with MAOIs may result in fatal reactions which includes hyperthermia, cardiovascular instability, autonomic instability, myoclonus and agitation progressing to delirium and coma. Thus, a minimum of 14 days after discontinuing therapy with the MAOI is required before initiating therapy with fluoxetine.
- **Liver impairment**: In patients with dysfunctional livers, doses of fluoxetine should be lowered in order to prevent drug accumulation in the plasma.
- **Kidney impairment**: In patients with dysfunctional kidneys, doses of fluoxetine should be lowered in order to prevent drug accumulation in the plasma.

Fluoxetine overdose

Fluoxetine overdose can be either un-intentional, or intentional.

The effects of fluoxetine overdose also depend on whether it was ingested alone or as a combination with other drugs and/ or with alcohol. As a general rule, the bigger the amount of fluoxetine ingested, the worse the reaction will get and the higher the possibility for lethal results.

General symptoms of fluoxetine overdose

Initially, the patient might feel extremely tired and lethargic. The pulse will slow down, and the breathing frequency will also reduce. As the level of intoxication increases, the level of consciousness will decrease, and the patient will become unresponsive to external stimulations.

The reflexes will disappear, and the breathing will get shallow. The patient's pulse and blood pressure will drop until cardiovascular system collapse.

Although fluoxetine **is relatively safe** and **rarely lethal in mono therapy overdose**, a combination of fluoxetine with alcohol and/ or with other central nervous depressants such as painkillers or benzo-diazepines may result in death caused by respiratory and cardiovascular depression.

The most common symptoms of fluoxetine over dose are

- nausea
- vomiting
- over sedation
- somnolence
- agitation
- abnormal heart rhythm: sinus tachycardia
- QTc prolongation

- dizziness
- sweating
- tremor
- convulsions
- amnesia
- confusion
- seizures
- cyanosis
- rabdomyolysis
- coma

What to do in the case of overdose

In general, there is no antidote for fluoxetine overdose. Management is mainly supportive, aimed at maintaining respiration, pulse and blood pressure.

In the event of a recent overdose with fluoxetine a stomach washout with activated charcoal might help in the elimination of the un-absorbed drug and is done with a large bore oro-gastric tube with appropriate airway protection. The aim of the stomach lavage is to get rid of the drug leftovers.

In some ER departments, ipecac is also used in order to induce vomiting of the ingested toxin, however **induction of emesis is not recommended in semi-comatose and comatose patients**.

Due to the large volume of distribution of fluoxetine, forced diuresis, dialysis hemo-perfusion and exchange transfusion are unlikely to be effective. Keeping open the patient's airway is compulsory, especially in semi - comatose individuals. The patient should be placed on his side in order to prevent aspiration of the vomitus back to the lungs. Suffocation due to vomit is the leading cause of death in fluoxetine overdose. Blood pressure and heart rate monitoring is very important. Fluid intake should be monitored with intra-venous infusion of saline and urinary output should be also carefully monitored. In most cases, fluoxetine overdose, requires hospitalization of the patient for at least 24 hours for intense observation.

Fluoxetine references

1 Akamine, Yumiko, Yasui-Furukori et al. Psychotropic drug – drug interactions involving P-gp. Nov 2012 Vol 26 issue 11- 959 – 973.

2 Weiss j, Dormann SM, Martin- Facklam et al. Inhibition of P-gp by newer antidepressants. J. Pharmacol Exp Ther. Apr 2003; 305(1):197-204.

3 Emslie G.J., Heiligenstein J., Wagner K.D, et al. Fluoxetine for acute treatment of depression in children and adolescent. J. of the American academy of child and adolescent psychiatry. 2002; 41, 1205-1215.

4 Becch P., Cialdella P, Haungh M, et al. Meta analysis of randomized controlled trials of fluoxetine versus placebo and TCA in the short term of MDD. J. of Psychiatry. 2000;176: 421-428.

5 Mcgareth PJ, Stewart J, Quitkin F, et al. Predictors of relapse in a prospective study of fluoxetine treatment of MDD. Am. J. Psychiatry 2006;163: 1542-1548.

6 Michelson D, Allgolacher C, Danlofer K et al. Efficacy of usual antidepressant regims of fluoxetine in panic disorder. B. J. of psychiatry 2001;179: 514-518.

12

Fluvoxamine

Brand name: Luvox

Mode of action of fluvoxamine

1 Fluvoxamine is a Serotonin Re-uptake Transporter *(SERT)* antagonist: The inhibition of the serotonin reuptake transporter (SERT), located on the presynaptic neurons, results in increased serotonin synaptic levels. In vivo, 50mg of fluvoxamine is able to occupy 72.9% - 76% of SERTs, suggesting that the starting dose of fluvoxamine is adequate to produce its clinical antidepressant effects.

2 *Sigma 1 receptors agonist:* The Sigma-1 receptor is a transmembrane protein, consisting of 223 amino acids and, produced in the endoplasmic reticulum. The sigma 1 receptor plays an important role in the regulation, and the modulation of the voltage-regulated and ligand- gated ion channels, which includes the $Ca(2+)$, $K+$, $Na+$, $Cl-$ and SK channels (1). In addition, the sigma- 1 receptor is involved in the inhibition of the voltage-gated K+ channels.

The sigma 1 receptor is also involved in the regulation of brain neurotransmitters which are involved in cell survival. It appears that sigma 1 agonism may promote neurogenesis and neural plasticity in several brain areas such as the prefrontal cortex, hipocampus and amygdala. The prefrontal cortex, hipocampus and amygdala are involved with stress, anxiety, depression and cognitive function impairment. Fluvoxamine is the only SSRI drug which has a strong affinity for the sigma 1 receptors, thus it has an important role in improving depression, anxiety, and other cognitive outcomes.

The selective effects of fluvoxamine on the anticholinergic, histaminergic and α adrenergic receptor are summarized as follows:

- ✓ **Anticholinergic Ach muscarinic affinity: Low.** Fluvoxamine has low incidence of side effects of dry mouth, constipation, blurred vision and drowsiness.

- ✓ **Histaminergic H1 affinity**: **Low.** Fluvoxamine has low incidence of side effects of sedation and weight gain.

- ✓ **α 1 adrenergic affinity**: **Low.** Fluvoxamine has low incidence of side effects of hypotension, dizziness, drowsiness and other cardiovascular effects.

Fluvoxamine's pharmacokinetics (Pk)

Fluvoxamine has **non-linear pharmacokinetics,** and it does inhibit its own metabolism. Each dose increase of fluvoxamine leads to a disproportionate increase in fluvoxamine plasma levels. Thus, the higher the daily dose of fluvoxamine, the disproportionately higher the plasma levels will get.

Peak plasma Time (tmax): 3-8 hours. Side effects of fluvoxamine are dose related and tend to emerge at the peak of its plasma level. A single dose of fluvoxamine may result in emerging side effects within 3 hours of drug ingestion.

Steady state: The daily use of fluvoxamine will reach a steady plasma level *within 7 days of* regular treatment.

Absorption: Fluvoxamine is well absorbed by the gastrointestinal system and its absorption is *not affected* by the presence of food.

Protein binding: 80%. Fluvoxamine is highly protein bound to albumin.

Half-Life (t 1/2): 15 hours. However, t 1/2 in the elderly can reach up to 25 hours.

Bioavailability: 53%

Distribution: 25L/kg

Fluvoxamine has an extensive tissue distribution. In addition to fluvoxamine's short half-life and lack of active metabolites, fluvoxamine has high lipid solubility, and small molecular size, which results in fluvoxamine easily crossing the blood-brain barrier, in a very high proportion.

Metabolism: Fluvoxamine is primarily metabolised by the liver enzymes CYP450: **3A4, 1A2, 2C9** and **2C19**.

Metabolites: Fluvoxamine has several **inactive metabolites**. Thus, due to its relative short half-life and the lack of therapeutic effect of its inactive metabolites, abrupt cessation of fluvoxamine may cause severe discontinuation symptoms.

Patients with liver disease can experience *a significant decrease* in fluvoxamine metabolism, which may result in increased fluvoxamine blood levels. Thus, patients with compromised livers require lower doses of fluvoxamine to avoid excessive accumulation of the drug in the blood.

Smokers may experience a 25% increase in fluvoxamine metabolism compared to non-smokers.

The P-gp system

Fluvoxamine is **an intermediate inhibitor of the P-gp functions** in vivo and in vitro (3,4). The inhibitory effects of fluvoxamine on the P-gp system might interfere with the plasma levels of other co-administered drugs, which are also P-gp substrates.

Elimination: Urine 94%. Fluvoxamine is eliminated mainly by the renal system. Thus, patients with renal impairment need to use fluvoxamine cautiously due to possible drug accumulation. Elderly patients >65 years may have 40% higher blood concentration of fluvoxamine as well as longer elimination half-life, which can reach up to 25.9 hours compared to a half-life of 15 hours in young patients.

How supplied

- Tablet: 25mg, 50mg, 100mg,
- Controlled released tablets (CR): 100mg and 150mg

Dose range

- 100 mg – 200 mg for depression
- 100mg – 300mg for OCD
- 100mg – 300mg for Social anxiety disorder.

Fluvoxamine clinical indications: US

- Obsessive compulsive disorder
- Social anxiety disorder

Indication outside the US

- Depression
- Obsessive compulsive disorder
- Social anxiety disorder
- Post Traumatic Stress Disorder
- Generalised anxiety disorder
- Panic disorder

Major Depressive Disorder (MDD)

Several studies have established the superiority of fluvoxamine over placebo in the treatment of major depression.

However, within the SSRI class, there is no evidence for superior effectiveness of one SSRI over another. In addition, there is no direct relationship between fluvoxamine's plasma concentration and the clinical response.

A double-blind randomised comparison study of fluvoxamine and fluoxetine conducted in an outpatients setting, on patients with MDD, randomized 184 patients to fluvoxamine 100mg/day or fluoxetine 20mg/day for 6 weeks. The study showed similar efficacy and response rates after 12 weeks of treatment as measured by HAMD-17items (5). Figure 10.3 shows fluvoxamine's response rates.

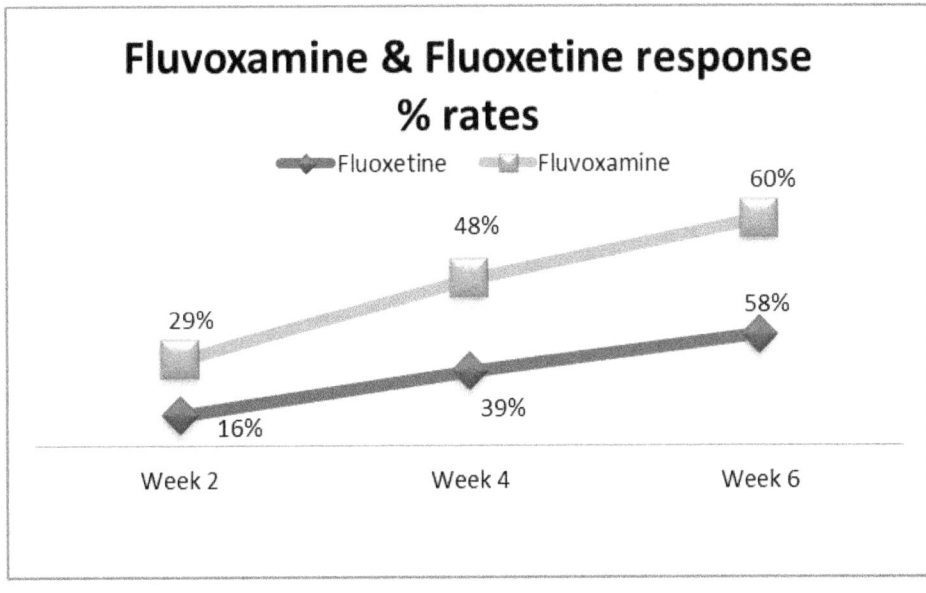

Figure 12.3: **Response rates of fluvoxamine compared to fluoxetine in MDD** Adapted from Dalery J, Honing A. Fluvoxamine versus Fluoxetine in MDD: A double-blind randomised comparison. Human Psychopharmacol Clin Exp 2003: 18:379-384 *(5).*

Furthermore, fluvoxamine has also shown to have long term efficacy in MDD (8).

Post traumatic stress disorder (PTSD)

Fluvoxamine was shown to be effective in the treatment of PTSD, both in the acute phase as well as in long term use.

Premenstrual Dysphoric Disorder (PMDD)

Fluvoxamine was shown to be effective in reducing the physical as well as the psychological symptoms of PMDD in doses up to 200mg a day.

Social anxiety disorder

Fluvoxamine is effective for the treatment of social anxiety disorder with an optimal daily dose of 200mg.

Generalized Anxiety Disorder (GAD)

Fluvoxamine was shown to be effective for the treatment of the acute phase of GAD as well as for long-term use at dose levels of 100 mg – 200 mg a day. The effects of fluvoxamine on GAD symptoms can last up to 6 months after the treatment is terminated.

Obsessive Compulsive Disorder (OCD)

Fluvoxamine also has been shown to be significantly effective for the treatment of Obsessive-Compulsive Disorder, independent of the patient's mood (9).

In a multicentre, randomized, double –blind, parallel group comparison study, 52% of the fluvoxamine-treated patient responded to a dose of 100mg -300mg, compared to only 18% of the placebo group (6).

In addition, fluvoxamine demonstrated long-term effects with a significant reduction in OCD relapse rate for up to 18 months (7).

The response and remission rates of fluvoxamine in OCD are illustrated in figure 12.2

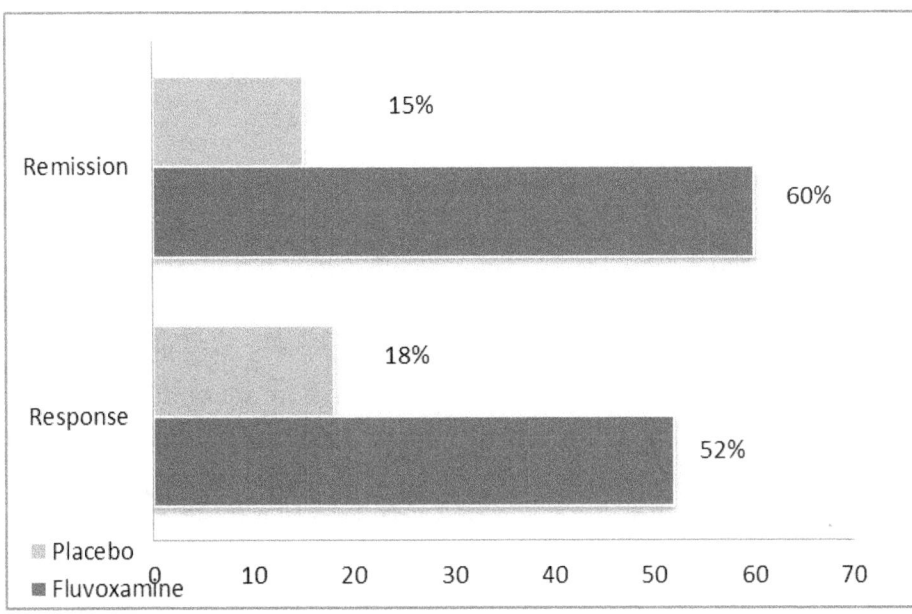

Figure 12.2 1: Response rate of fluvoxamine and placebo in OCD patients adapted from Figgit DP, McClellan KJ. Fluvoxamine: an update review of its use in the management of adults with anxiety disorders. Drugs 2000;60(4): 925-954. *(6).* **2 The long term remission study with fluvoxamine and placebo in OCD patients.** *A*dapted from Ravizza L, Barzega G, Bellino S. Drug treatment of obsessive-compulsive disorder (OCD): long-term trial with clomipramine and selective serotonin reuptake inhibitors. Psychopharmacol Bull. 1996;32:167-73. *(7).*

Panic disorder (PD)

Although the currently available data suggests that the effective dose of fluvoxamine for PD, is 100 mg a day, inter-patient variation shows that some individuals may require a lower dose.

The overall duration of treatment with fluvoxamine for panic disorder is 6–12 months. However, in some cases a longer period of treatment is required, possibly indefinitely.

How to treat with Fluvoxamine

- **For Major Depression (MDD):** Start with 50mg a day in a single morning dose. Wait at least one week to assess clinical improvement before increasing the dose in increments of 50mg a day to a maximum of 200mg a day. With the CR formulation, start with initial dose of 100mg a day to be increased by 50 mg/day weekly up to a maximum of 200mg/day, if needed.

- **For OCD:** Start with 50mg a day to be increased weekly up to a maximum of 300mg a day if required.

- **For Panic disorder, Social anxiety and PMDD:** as for depression.

As a general rule, the higher the patient's anxiety is, the lower the starting dose should be and the slower the dose increase should be in order to minimize the risk of activation.

When and how to take fluvoxamine

Preferably take fluvoxamine at night.

How to stop fluvoxamine

Due to its short half-life, and the potential to develop withdrawal syndrome, a slow tapering of fluvoxamine is highly recommended.

The patient must reduce the dose of fluvoxamine gradually by a rate of 50% every 3 days. In the case of getting withdrawal symptoms, re-instate the previous dose. Once the symptoms disappear, start reducing the fluvoxamine dose in smaller proportions and over a longer period. In cases of acute withdrawal symptoms, add an SSRI with a longer half-life such as fluoxetine in order to avoid serious withdrawal symptoms. Only then stop fluvoxamine and thereafter, fluoxetine can be slowly reduced without the risk of getting discontinuation symptoms.

How long it takes to get antidepressant effects with fluvoxamine

In order to get an antidepressant effect, fluvoxamine should be used daily for at least 2 – 4 weeks. Fluvoxamine's efficacy can increase by increasing the dose, as many patients experience a beneficial antidepressant effect with a daily dose of 200 mg of fluvoxamine. Like all antidepressants, fluvoxamine requires time before a substantial mood improvement can be evident.

Side effects of Fluvoxamine

Most side effects of fluvoxamine are related to the serotonin increase in the brain as well as in other body parts. Most side effects develop soon after the initiation of treatment and often disappear with time. The most common side effects of fluvoxamine are:

Nervous system

- Agitation

- Restlessness
- Jitteriness
- anxiety
- Tremor
- increased sweating
- flushing
- headache
- dizziness
- seizures (rare)
- somnolence
- cognitive slowing
- reduced attention
- apathy
- emotional blunting
- rash

Gastro intestinal (GI)

The gastro intestinal side effects can develop within 30 minutes of drug ingestion, and they are more likely the result of the direct effect of fluvoxamine on the intestinal mucosa than the plasma peak level.

- decreased appetite
- upper gastrointestinal symptoms
- nausea
- vomiting
- dry mouth
- diarrhea
- constipation
- Possible weight loss

Sexual

The incidence of the sexual side effects attributed to all the SSRIs is approximately between 20% - 40% of treated patients.

The sexual side effects of fluvoxamine are dose-dependent and do not diminish over time.

The most common fluvoxamine sexual side effects are:

- decreased sex drive
- delayed ejaculation
- impotence
- inability to reach an orgasm

Suicide

The FDA requires all antidepressants to carry a black box warning stating that antidepressants may increase the risk for suicide in persons under the age of 25 years. This warning is based on data suggesting that suicidal ideations and behavior have a 2 fold increase in children and in adolescents, and a 1.5 - fold increase in the 18 - 24 age group.

Side effect that need immediate attention:

- Confusion
- Excitation
- Onset of seizure
- Yellow skin / yellow eyes
- Severe allergic reaction
- Irregular heart beats
- Low blood pressure
- Bruising and bleeding(relatively rare)
- Induction of manic episode
- Activation of suicidal ideation and behaviour

Physical & psychological dependence

Fluvoxamine did not show any tendencies for drug seeking behaviour.

However, patients with a history of drug abuse should be closely monitored for signs of fluvoxamine misuse or abuse, which include drug seeking behavior, development of tolerance and dose incrementations.

Fluvoxamine discontinuation reaction

The most common symptoms of sudden discontinuation offluvoxamine are:

- Nausea
- Stomach cramps
- Sweating
- tingling
- dizziness
- light-handedness
- vertigo
- feeling of electricity in the body
- anxiety

Safety profile of fluvoxamine

Use in pregnancy: Risk category C

Fluvoxamine is classified by the FDA as having a risk category C.

The risk of pregnant mothers with a history of depression to develop depression during their pregnancy and especially after child delivery is very high and often requires the continuation of the treatment with SSRIs during and after the pregnancy.

In addition, the use of fluvoxamine in the last trimester of pregnancy is associated with higher incidence of respiratory distress and pulmonary hypertension, cyanosis, apnea, seizures, temperature instability, vomiting, hypoglycemia, hypotonia, hyperreflexia, tremor, irritability, constant crying and jitteriness, and subsequent prolonged hospitalization, tube feeding and respiratory support. There is an increased risk of the newborn developing PPHN associated with substantial neonatal morbidity and mortality. The risk of developing PPHN was six-fold higher in infants exposed to SSRIs after the 20th week of gestation. It appears that the risk of getting PPHN is common in all the SSRI medications used during the pregnancy. Thus, the use of fluvoxamine during the first trimester as well as throughout the pregnancy is not recommended.

Use during lactation

Fluvoxamine is secreted in the breast milk. Due to its unknown effects on the new born's normal growth and development, breast feeding should be avoided.

Carcinogenesis

There is no evidence of carcinogenesis, mutagenicity or impaired fertility with fluvoxamine. Treatment of rats for 30 months at doses of fluvoxamine, 6 times the maximum human daily dose, did not cause any carcinogenicity. In addition, treatment of rats at doses of fluvoxamine, 2 times the maximum human daily dose, had no effect on mating performance, duration of gestation or pregnancy.

Fluvoxamine drug interaction

Follow a list of fluvoxamine drug interaction with concomitant medication

- **Warfarin**: the concomitant use may Increase in warfarin blood levels which carries the risk of bleeding.
- **Carbamazepine**: The concomitant use may Increased carbamazepine blood levels which may cause symptoms of carbamazepine toxicity.
- **MAOI:** The concomitant use may cause CNS toxicity - serotonin syndrome. Wait 21 days after MAOI was stopped before initiating treatment with fluvoxamine. Wait 7 days to start MAOI after discontinuing fluvoxamine.
- **Alprazolam & Triazolam:** The concomitant use may Increased alprazolam & triazolam blood levels.
- Buspirone: The concomitant use may cause a **3-fold increase** in buspirone plasma levels.
- Statines: The concomitant use may Increased statin blood levels.
- Clozapine, Pimozide & Thioridazine: The concomitant use may Increased plasma levels of clozapine & Pimozide & thioridazine, which may cause QTc prolongation and cardiac arrhythmias.
- **Caffeine & Teophilline**: The concomitant use may Increased caffeine blood levels (the caffeine half-life may increase from 5 hours to 30 hours). Increasing symptoms of anxiety and jitteriness and also possibly causing seizure.
- **Propranolol & Metoprolol**: The concomitant use may Increased propranolol & metoprolol blood levels 5–fold. Such increases in the betablocker blood levels may enhance bradycardia and lethargy.
- **Tramadol**: The concomitant use may cause seizure.
- **Sildenafil;** The concomitant use may Increased sildenafil blood levels which may increase the possibility of low blood pressure.
- **Sumatrip**tan: The concomitant use may cause weakness and in-coordination.

- **Methadone:** The concomitant use may significantly increase methadone levels which may cause symptoms of methadone intoxication.

Warnings for fluvoxamine

> **Pregnancy: Risk category** C. Triy to avoid use during pregnancy or breastfeeding. Assessment of the risks versus benefits must be discussed with the patient.
> **Fluvoxamine may cause an increase in suicidal risk in young adults.** Pooled analysis of trials of drugs used for MDD showed that SNRIs and SSRIs may increase the risk of suicidal thinking and behavior in children, adolescents and young adults aged 18-24. The use of antidepressants in this population must balance the risk of suicide with the clinical need. Careful monitoring of the patient's clinical worsening and suicidality should also involve the family and all other caregivers.
> **Fluvoxamine** may cause **serotonin syndrome**
> **Activation of hypomania or mania** occurred in 1% of fluvoxamine-treated bipolar patients. As fluvoxamine may trigger mania in predisposed patients, it should be used cautiously in patients with a history of bipolar mood disorder.
> **Hyponatremia** may develop subsequent to the use of fluvoxamine, especially in volume depleted patients and in patients on diuretics. It is possible that hyponatremia results from the syndrome of inappropriate antidiuretic hormone secretion (SIADH). The symptoms of hyponatremia include headaches, reduced concentration, confusion, weakness and unsteadiness, which may lead to falls. Severe cases of hyponatremia may result in seizures, hallucinations, respiratory arrest, coma and death. Elderly patients appear to be at a higher risk. Fluvoxamine discontinuation often results in symptom resolution.

- **Abnormal bleeding** was observed in patients using fluvoxamine. Concomitant use of warfarin, NSAIDs and aspirin along with fluvoxamine may add to this risk.
- **The incidence of seizures** occurred only in 0.2% of fluvoxamine-treated patients. Fluvoxamine should be used cautiously in patients with a history of seizures.
- **Withdrawal reaction.** Fluvoxamine may cause withdrawal reaction. Prevention of withdrawal necessitates a slow reduction of fluvoxamine doses. The onset of withdrawal symptoms is attributed to fluvoxamine's short half-life as well as to the lack of active metabolite. The withdrawal symptoms of fluvoxamine can develop as early as the second day of the drug's sudden discontinuation and may persist for several days. The most common withdrawal symptoms are nausea, dizziness, insomnia, anxiety, and headache.
- **Liver dysfunction.** Fluvoxamine requires dose reduction in patients with liver dysfunction due to its extensive metabolism by the liver CYP 450 enzymatic system.
- **Kidney dysfunction.** Fluvoxamine requires a lower dose in patients with kidney impairment due to its elimination in the urine.
- **Elderly.** Fluvoxamine requires lower dose in the elderly due to a longer half-life in patients above 65 years.
- **MAOI.** Fluvoxamine requires a **two-week washout period** before starting with MAOI and one week washout period before changing from MAOI to fluvoxamine..
- **Alcohol.** The patient should be advised to **avoid alcohol** while taking fluvoxamine.

Overdose

Fluvoxamine overdose can be either un-intentional, or intentional. The effects of fluvoxamine overdose also depend whether it was ingested alone or as a combination with other drugs and/ or with alcohol. As a general rule, the bigger the amount of fluvoxamine ingested, the worse the reaction will get and rhe higher the possibility for lethal results.

General symptoms of fluvoxamine overdose:

Initially, the patient might feel extremely tired and lethargic. The pulse will slow down, and the breathing frequency will also decrease. As the level of intoxication increases, the level of consciousness will decrease, and the patient will become unresponsive to external stimulations. The reflexes will disappear, and the breathing will get shallow. The patient's pulse and blood pressure will drop until cardiovascular system collapse.

Although fluvoxamine **is relatively safe** and **rarely lethal in mono therapy overdose**, a combination of fluvoxamine with alcohol and/ or with other central nervous system depressants such as painkillers or benzo-diazepines may result in death cause by respiratory and cardiovascular depression.

Symptoms of fluvoxamine over dose are

- vomiting
- over sedation
- somnolence
- agitation
- dizziness
- diarrhea
- abnormal heart rhythm
- tachycardia
- bradycardia
- hypokalemia
- hypotension
- nausea
- respiratory difficulties

- tremor
- convulsion
- coma

What to do in the case of overdose

In general, there is no antidote for fluvoxamine overdose. Management is mainly supportive, aimed at maintaining respiration, pulse and blood pressure.

In the event of a recent overdose with fluvoxamine a stomach washout with activated charcoal might help in the elimination of the un-absorbed drug and is done with a large bore oro-gastric tube with appropriate airway protection. The aim of the stomach lavage is to get rid of the drug leftovers.

In some ER departments, ipecac is also used in order to induce vomiting of the ingested toxin, however **induction of emesis is not recommended in semi-comatose and comatose patients**. Due to the large volume of distribution of fluvoxamine, forced diuresis, dialysis hemo-perfusion and exchange transfusion are unlikely to be effective. Keeping open the patient's airway is compulsory, especially in semi - comatose individuals. The patient should be placed on his side in order to prevent aspiration of the vomitus back to the lungs. Suffocation due to vomit is the leading cause of death in fluvoxamine overdose. Blood pressure and heart rate monitoring is very important. Fluid intake should be monitored with intra -venous infusion of saline and urinary output should be also carefully monitored. In most cases, fluvoxamine overdose, requires hospitalization of the patient for at least 24 hours for intense observation.

Fluvoxamine reference

1 Ther P, . The pharmacology of sigma – 1 receptors. Pharmacol Ther, November 2009; 124(2): 195-206.

2 Akamine, Yumiko,Yasui-Furukori et al. Psychotropic drug – drug interactions involving P-gp. Nov 2012 Vol 26 issue 11- 959 – 973.

3 Weiss j, Dormann SM, Martin- Facklam et al. Inhibition of P-gp by newer antidepressants. J. Pharmacol Exp Ther. Ap 2003; 305(1):197-204.

4. Yasui- Furukori N, Takahta T, Nakaguri T. Different inhibitory effects of fluvoxamine on omeprazole . Br. J. Clin. Pharmacology, April 2004;57 (4) 487 – 494.

5 Dalery J, Honing A. Fluvoxamine versus Fluoxetine in MDD: A double-blind randomised comparison. Human Psychopharmacol Clin Exp 2003: 18:379-384.

6 Figgit DP, McClellan KJ,. Fluvoxamine: an update review of its use in the management of adults with anxiety disorders. Drugs, 2000; 60(4): 925-954.

7 Ravizza L, Barzega G, Bellino S. Drug treatment of obsessive-compulsive disorder (OCD): long-term trial with clomipramine and selective serotonin reuptake inhibitors (SSRIs)Psychopharmacol Bull. 1996;32:167–73.

8 Martin AJ, Wakelin J,. Fluvoxamine: a baseline study of clinical response, long term tolerance and safety in a general practice population. Br J Clin Pract 40-:95-99, 1986.

9 Freeman CP, Trimble MR, Deakin JFW et al: Fluvoxamine versus clomipramine in the treatment of OCD: a multicentre, randomized, double –blind, paralled group cpmparison. J Clin Psychiatry 1994;55(7): 301-305.

13

Imipramine

Brand names:

Tofranil

Deprinol

Depsonil

Dynaprin

Imipramil

Imipramine's Mode of Action

1. Imipramine is a potent SERT <u>antagonist</u>. The inhibition of the Serotonin Reuptake Transporter, located on the presynaptic neurons, results in increased serotonin synaptic levels. The inhibition of SERT by imipramine is as strong as that of SSRIs.

2. Desipramine (imipramine's active metabolite) is a potent <u>antagonist</u> of the Norepinephrine Reuptake Transporter *(NET)*: The inhibition of the presynaptic norepinephrine reuptake transporter results in increased norepinephrine synaptic levels.

The selective effects of imipramine on the anticholinergic, histaminergic and α adrenergic receptor are summarized as follows:

- ✓ **Anticholinergic Ach muscarinic affinity: High.** Imipramine has high incidence of side effects of dry mouth, constipation, blurred vision and drowsiness.

- ✓ **Histaminergic H1 affinity**: **High**. Imipramine has a high incidence of side effects of sedation and weight gain.

- ✓ **α 1 adrenergic affinity**: **High**. Imipramine has a high incidence of side effects of hypotension, dizziness, drowsiness and other cardiovascular effects.

Imipramine Pharmacokinetics

Imipramine has **linear pharmacokinetics**. Thus any dose change leads to a proportional change in the drug plasma levels. However, in overdose, nonlinear kinetics is more likely to occur.

Peak plasma levels (t max): 2-8 hours. Imipramine's side effects are related and tend to emerge at the peak of its plasma level. A single dosing of imipramine may result in emerging side effects within 2 hours after drug ingestion.

It appears that there is a relationship between imipramine plasma level and clinical response. Imipramine plasma levels >200ng/mL result in increased efficacy.

For imipramine's active metabolite, *desipramine*, effective plasma levels are those above 125ng/mL. Plasma levels above 300ng/mL result in higher toxicity for both imipramine and desipramine. The risk for atrioventricular block is higher at imipramine plasma concentrations > 350ng/mL (5).

Absorption: Imipramine is well absorbed by the gastrointestinal system, mainly in the small intestine. It is not affected by the presence of food. Imipramine is a basic lipophilic amine that distributes throughout the body with a high volume of distribution. Imipramine's concentration in the cardiac tissue is higher than that in the plasma.

Bioavailability: Unknown

Protein bounding: **>90%.** Imipramine is highly protein bound. More than 98% of the circulating imipramine is attached to the plasma proteins, albumin and α1-glycoprotein.

Imipramine elimination half- life (t 1/2): 5-30 hours for the parent drug. The longer half-life of imipramine's metabolite **desipramine** results in a lower risk of discontinuation symptoms and a higher risk of drug interaction.

Steady state: Imipramine reaches a steady state concentration within **5-7 days** of regular use.

Metabolism: Imipramine is primarily metabolised by the liver via the enzymes CYP450: **2D6 and 1A2.**

Hepatic metabolism occurs via demethylation of the side chain and via hydroxylation of the ring structure into hydroxyl metabolites. The plasma levels of 2-hydroxydesipramine is 50% of that of the parent drug (6).

The active metabolite of imipramine is called *desipramine* which has a strong affinity for the presynaptic Norepinephrine Reuptake Transporters (NET).

The P-gp System

Imipramine is an **inhibitor** of the P-gp system (3).

Elimination: Urine >80%

How imipramine is supplied

- Capsules of 75mg, 125mg, 150mg
- Tablets 10mg, 25mg, 50 mg,

Dose range

- Imipramine 50mg -300mg a day for depression

Imipramine Clinical indications

- Major depression
- Enuresis (involuntary nightly urination during sleep) in children and adolescents.
- Anxiety
- Neuropathic pain
- Insomnia
- Treatment resistant depression
- Cataplexy syndrome

Chronic pain syndrome

Imipramine is used for chronic pain and migraine headaches prophylaxis.

Enuresis & Premature ejaculation

Imipramine, like other TCA medications, is highly effective in preventing involuntary night time urination during sleep as well as in delaying ejaculation during sexual intercourse. It is believed that the anticholinergic side effects of imipramine are responsible for its beneficial effects in these two conditions. For enuresis the dose of imipramine is 25mg–50mg at bedtime.

Major Depressive Disorder (MDD)

The efficacy of imipramine in the treatment of depression showed comparable efficacy to that of other tricyclic antidepressants. In a prospective comparative study of 60 patients randomized to be treated with moclobemide or imipramine for a period of 6 weeks, both groups showed a significant decrease in HAM-D scores at the end of 6 weeks (4).

Imipramine at a full dose is also effective for depression maintenance. In a three-year follow up study (7), imipramine maintained its efficacy in 80% of the depressed patients compared to 10% of patients on placebo. Figure 13.1 illustrates these results.

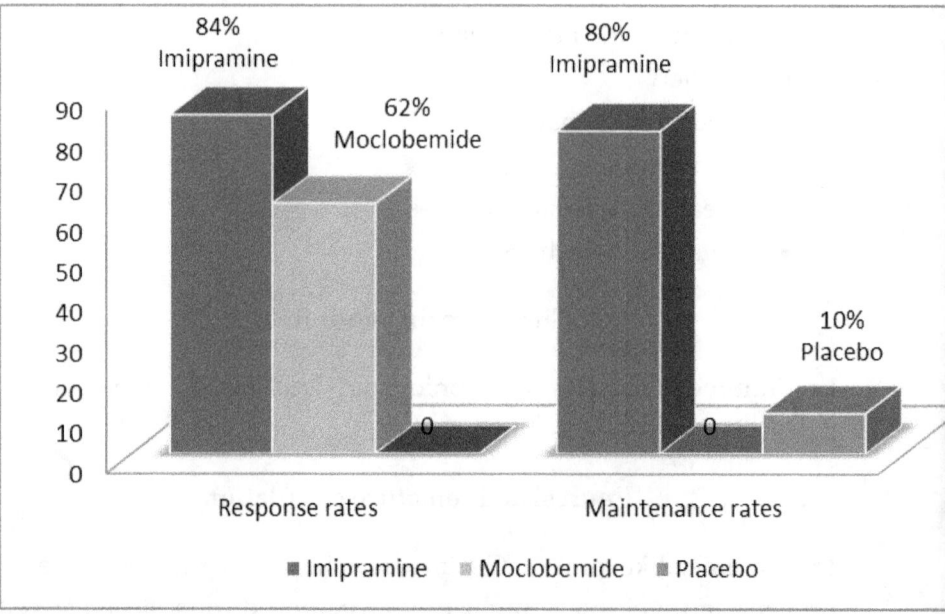

Figure 13.1: Imipramine and Moclobemide response rates in the treatment of MDD. Adapted from response study by A Avanti, P Kulhare,G Singh et al. Comparison of the efficacy and safety of moclobemide and imipramine in the treatment of depression in Indian patients. India J of Psychiatry. 2005 47 (2) 84-88. And from a maintenance study by E Frank, DJ Kupfer, JM Perel, et al. Three - years outcome for maintenance therapies in recurrent depression. Arch Gen Psychiatry, 1990, 47:1093-1099.

Although the FDA approved the use of imipramine only for the treatment of major depression, imipramine is also used for enuresis, insomnia, anxiety and neuropathic pain.

How to treat with imipramine

- **For Major Depression (MDD):** start imipramine with 25mg preferably at bedtime and slowly increase the dose by increments of 25mg every 3 days to a maximum of 300mg taken at bedtime in order to avoid daily sedation.

When and how to take medication:

Preferably take imipramine at bedtime to avoid over sedation. In general, "start low and go slow", as patients can experience over-sedation the following day at the beginning of the treatment.

How to stop imipramine

It is highly recommended to slow taper imipramine in order to minimize the emergence of withdrawal symptoms, which usually develop within the first 2 weeks of treatment cessation. Imipramine requires a gradual dose reduction in order to avoid discontinuation symptoms.

A 50% dose reduction every third day is recommended. In the event of the patient developing withdrawal symptoms, re instate the previous dose. Once the symptoms disappear, start reducing the imipramine dose in lower proportions and over a longer period of time.

How long it takes to get an antidepressant effect

Like all antidepressants, imipramine needs at least 7–28 days before a substantial mood improvement emerges.

Imipramine side effects

Most side effects of imipramine are probably related to its ability to increase serotonin in the brain, as well as its inhibitory effects on the $\alpha 1$ adrenergic receptors and the H1 histaminergic receptors, often resulting in hypotension and over-sedation. Most side effects are usually dose related and often develop soon after the initiation of treatment, and subside with time. The most common side effects of imipramine are:

Nervous system

- numbness
- paresthesis of extremities
- incoordination
- ataxia
- extrapyramidal symptoms
- drowsiness
- lethargy
- fatigue
- weakness
- dizziness
- insomnia
- nausea
- blurred vision
- headache and worsening of migraine
- in coordination
- tremor
- disturbed concentration
- disorientation
- confusion
- restlessness and agitation (rare)
- *seizures*.
- stuttering
- disturbance in gait
- worsening of parkinsonism
- rush (rare)
- hypotension
- syncope
- bradycardia

Gastro intestinal

The gastro intestinal side effects can develop within 30 minutes of drug ingestion, and they are more likely the result of imipramine's effects on serotonin uptake and its anticholinergic effects.

- *decreased appetite*
- *heartburn*
- **weight gain (up to 18% of treated patients)**
- nausea
- vomiting
- dry mouth
- constipation
- gastritis
- diarrhea
- peculiar taste
- black tongue
- stomatitis
- abdominal cramps
- epigastric distress
- anorexia

Sexual

- decreased libido
- impotence
- retrograde ejaculation
- painful ejaculation
- delayed ejaculation

Endocrine

- gynecomastia in males
- galactorrhea in female

- breast enlargement in females
- testicular swelling
- Syndrome of inappropriate antidiuretic hormone (SIADH).

Hematologic

- thrombocytopenia
- purpura
- eosinophilia
- agranulocytosis

Allergic

- skin rash
- urticarial
- itching
- photosensitization
- edema
- cross sensitivity with desipramine

Suicide

The FDA requires all antidepressants to carry a black box warning stating that antidepressants may increase the risk for suicide in persons under the age of 25 years. This warning is based on data suggesting that suicidal ideations and behavior has a 2-fold increase in children and in adolescents, and a 1.5 – fold increase in the 18 – 24 age group.

Imipramine side effect that require immediate attention

- Confusion
- Excitation
- Onset of seizure
- Yellow skin / eyes

- Severe allergic reaction
- Irregular heart beats
- Hypotension
- Induction of manic or hypomanic episode
- Activation of suicidal ideation and behaviour especially in children and adolescents

Physical & psychological dependence

Imipramine did not show any tendencies for drug seeking behaviour. However, patients with a history of drug abuse should be closely monitored for signs of imipramine misuse or abuse, which include drug seeking behavior, development of tolerance and unwarranted dose increases.

Imipramine discontinuation reaction

Sudden discontinuation of imipramine may be associated with a discontinuation reaction.

The discontinuation symptoms are usually self-limiting. The most common symptoms of discontinuation reaction are:

- irritability
- agitation
- dizziness
- anxiety
- confusion
- headache
- lethargy
- insomnia
- seizures
- dysphoric mood
- fever
- fatigue
- sweating

- myalgia (muscle pain)

A slow down-titration of imipramine may reduce the risk of developing a discontinuation reaction.

Safety profile of imipramine

Use in pregnancy: FDA risk category D

According the FDA imipramine is **risk category D** (positive evidence of risk to human fetus however, there have been no well – controlled studies with pregnant women). The risk of pregnant mothers with a history of depression to develop depression during their pregnancy and especially after child delivery is very high and often requires the continuation of the treatment with SSRIs during and after the pregnancy.

There were clinical reports of congenital malformations associated with the use of imipramine during pregnancy. Furthermore, the use of imipramine, like with all antidepressants, in the last trimester is associated with higher incidence of respiratory distress and pulmonary hypertension, cyanosis, apnea, seizures, temperature instability vomiting, hypoglycemia, hypotonia, hyperreflexia, tremor, irritability, constant crying and jitteriness with subsequent prolonged hospitalization, tube feeding and respiratory support. There is an increased risk of the newborn to developing PPHN and it is associated with substantial neonatal morbidity and mortality. Thus, the use of imipramine during the first trimester as well as throughout the pregnancy is not recommended.

Use during lactation:

Imipramine is secreted in human breast milk. Due to its unknown effects on the newborn's normal growth and development breast feeding should be avoided.

Carcinogenesis

There is no evidence of carcinogenesis, teratogenicity, mutagenicity or impaired fertility with imipramine use.

Avoid using imipramine in the following cases

- **Myocardial infarction:** Patients recovering from myocardial infarction should avoid using imipramine due to its propensity to cause cardiac arrhythmias, heart block, prolongation of conduction time, hypotension and worsening of congestive heart failure.
- **Hyperthyroidism** Patients with hyperthyroidism are more sensitive to imipramine's side effects.
- **Cardiac arrhythmia:** Patients with pre-existing cardiac disease and cardiac arrhythmias should be closely monitored and preferably avoid the use of imipramine.
- **History of seizure**
- **Prostate hypertrophy**
- **Pre-existing closed angle glaucoma due to imipramine's anticholinergic effects.**
- **Proven allergy to imipramine.**

Follows a list of imipramine drug interactions:

- **Warfarin:** The concomitant use may Increased PT time.
- **Carbamazepine:** The concomitant use may Decreases imipramine plasma levels due to P450 liver enzyme induction by carbamazepine.
- **Antiarrhytmic:** The concomitant use may cause prolongation of cardiac conduction.
- **Phenobarbital:** The concomitant use may Increased phenobarbital plasma levels.
- **Akineton:** The concomitant use may Increased overall anticholinergic effects.

- **Fluoxetine & Paroxetine &Duloxetine & Bupropion**: The concomitant use may Increase imipramine plasma levels.
- **Ketoconazole**: The concomitant use may Increased imipramine plasma levels.
- **MAOI**: The concomitant use may cause CNS toxicity-serotonin syndrome. Patients must wait 21 days after MAOI was stopped before initiating treatment with imipramine. Patient must wait 5-7 days to start MAOI after discontinuing imipramine.
- **Methylphenidate**: The concomitant use **may Increased** imipramine plasma levels.
- **Fluvoxamine**: The concomitant use **may Increased** imipramine plasma concentration.
- **Grapefruit juice:** The concomitant use **may decreased** imipramine metabolism due to inhibition of the liver enzyme **3A4** by the grapefruit juice which results in increased imipramine blood levels.
- **Tamoxifen:** The concomitant use **may decreased** imipramine plasma levels.
- **Triptans:** The concomitant use may cause serotonergic reaction.

Warnings for imipramine:

> **Pregnancy**: **Risk category D**. Try to avoid use during pregnancy or breastfeeding. Assessment of the risks versus benefits must be discussed with the patient.
> **Seizure risk**. Imipramine doses higher than 300mg are associated with increased risk of seizure. Thus caution should be used in administration of imipramine to patients with a history of seizure and to patients with other predisposing factors such as brain damage, and in alcohol abusers.

> **Imipramine may cause an increase in suicidal risk in young adults.** Pooled analysis of trials of drugs used for MDD showed that SNRIs and SSRIs may increase the risk of suicidal thinking and behavior in children, adolescents and young adults aged 18-24. The use of any antidepressant in this population must balance the risk of suicide with the clinical need. Careful monitoring of the patient's clinical worsening, and suicidality should also involve the family and all other caregivers cause increases in suicidal risk in young adults.
> **Activation of hypomania or mania** may occur in imipramine-treated bipolar patients. As imipramine may trigger mania in predisposed patients, it should be used cautiously in patients with a history of bipolar mood disorder
> **Serotonin syndrome** may develop with imipramine use. Serotonin syndrome symptoms may include agitation, dizziness, hallucinations, delirium, seizures and coma along with autonomic instability which includes tachycardia, fluctuating blood pressure, flushing, hyperthermia, tremor, muscular rigidity, myoclonus, hyperreflexia, and incoordination. The concomitant use of imipramine with MAOIs, triptans, TCAs, Lithium, fentanyl, tramadol, tryptophan, buspirone and St. John's Wort may precipitate serotonin syndrome.
> **Cardiac impairment:** Imipramine needs to be used with caution in patients with cardiac impairment. Imipramine use was associated with low blood pressure, ECG abnormalities including ST-T wave changes, PVCs and intraventricular conduction abnormalities. An ECG should be recorded prior to treatment initiation with imipramine.
> **S/P MI:** Imipramine should be avoided in patients who recently had a myocardial infarct.

- **Renal impairment**: Imipramine requires lower dose in mild to moderate renal impairment.
- **Liver impairment**: Imipramine must be avoided in patients with liver insufficiency.
- **Alcohol:** Imipramine is not recommended in patients abusing alcohol.
- **Withdrawal reaction.** Imipramine use may cause withdrawal reaction, which can be avoided by a slow reduction of imipramine doses. The onset of withdrawal symptoms is attributed to imipramine's relative short half-life. The withdrawal symptoms of imipramine can develop as early as the second day of the sudden discontinuation, and may persist for several days. The most common withdrawal symptoms are nausea, dizziness, insomnia, anxiety, tension and headache.
- **Narrow-angel glaucoma**: Imipramine use in patients with glaucoma may be associated with increased intraocular pressure due to it anticholinergic properties.
- **Urinary retention**: Imipramine may worsen urinary retention in predisposed patients due to its anticholinergic properties.
- **Hyperthyroidism:** Imipramine's cardiac toxicity may be increased in patients with hyperthyroidism or patients on thyroid medications.
- **Adrenal medulla tumors:** Imipramine use in patients with adrenal tumors such as pheochromocytoma or neuroblastoma may be associated with hypertensive crisis.
- **MAOI:** Imipramine's combined use with MAOI might be fatal. Imipramine requires a **7 day** washout period before starting with a MAOI, and a **3 week** washout period after the MAOI was stopped before starting with imipramine.
- **Elderly:** Imipramine needs a lower dose in the elderly. Elderly patients with cardiac disease are at special risk of developing cardiac abnormalities.

- ➤ **Weight**: Imipramine may be associated with weight gain.
- ➤ **Hematologic changes**: Imipramine may be associated with leukopenia, agranulocytosis, thrombocytopenia, anemia, and pancytopenia. Leukocyte and a differential blood count should be obtained immediately in patients who develop fever and sore throat.
- ➤ **Hyperthermia**: Imipramine may be associated with hyperthermia, especially when it was used in combination with other drugs.
- ➤ **ECT**: The concurrent use of imipramine with ECT may increase the cardiac related hazards of ECT.

Imipramine overdose

Imipramine overdose can be either un-intentional, or intentional.

The effects of imipramine overdose also depend whether it was ingested alone or as a combination with other drugs and/ or with alcohol. As a general rule, the bigger the amount of imipramine ingested, the worse the reaction will get and the higher the possibility for lethal results.

Symptoms of imipramine overdose

Initially, the patient might feel extremely tired and lethargic. The pulse will slow down, and the breathing frequency will also decrease. As the level of intoxication increases, the level of consciousness will decrease, and the patient will become unresponsive to external stimulations. The reflexes will disappear, and the breathing will get shallow. The patient's pulse and blood pressure will drop until cardiovascular system collapse.

Imipramine may be lethal in mono therapy overdose as it has a high incidence of fatalities. In addition, the concomitant use of imipramine with alcohol and with other central nervous system depressants such as painkillers or benzo- diazepines may result in death caused by respiratory depression. The possible fatalities are often the result of cardio-respiratory arrest, or with the metabolic acidosis and hypoxia associated with status epilepticus.

Symptoms of imipramine over dose are

- over sedation
- drowsiness
- respiratory depression
- cyanosis
- respiratory arrest
- seizure
- abnormal heart rhythm – mainly tachycardia
- ECG changes – in QRS axis
- congestive heart failure
- cardiac arrest
- hypotension
- hyperactive reflexes
- muscle rigidity
- coreiform movements
- mydriasis
- oliguria
- anuria
- vomiting
- delirium
- disorientation
- hallucinations
- delusions
- anxiety
- restlessness
- agitation
- loss of consciousness

What to do in the case of overdose

In general, there is no antidote for imipramine overdose. Management is mainly supportive, aimed at maintaining respiration, pulse and blood pressure. In the event of a recent overdose with imipramine a stomach washout with activated charcoal might help in the elimination of the un-absorbed drug and is done with a large bore oro-gastric tube with appropriate airway protection. The aim of the stomach lavage is to get rid of the drug leftovers.

In some ER departments, ipecac is also used in order to induce vomiting of the ingested toxin, however **induction of emesis is not recommended in semi-comatose and comatose patients.**

Due to the large volume of distribution of imipramine, forced diuresis, dialysis hemo-perfusion and exchange transfusion are unlikely to be effective.

Keeping open the patient's airway is compulsory, especially in semi - comatose individuals. The patient should be placed on his side in order to prevent aspiration of the vomitus back to the lungs. Suffocation due to vomit is the leading cause of death in imipramine overdose. Blood pressure and heart rate monitoring is very important. **There are several case reports of death following imipramine overdose due to a fatal arrhythmia which develops a day after overdose.** Imipramine plasma level should not guide patient's management. QRS duration of >0.10 second may be the best indication of the severity of imipramine overdose. I.V sodium bicarbonate should be used to keep plasma pH in the range of 7.45 – 7.55. Fluid intake should be monitored with intra-venous infusion of saline and urinary output should be also carefully monitored. In most cases, imipramine overdose, requires hospitalization of the patient for at least 24 hours for intense observation.

Imipramine references

1 Akamine, Yumiko,Yasui-Furukori et al. Psychotropic drug – drug interactions involving P-gp. Nov 2012 Vol 26 issue 11- 959 – 973.

2 Weiss j, Dormann SM, Martin- Facklam et al. Inhibition of P-gp by newer antidepressants. J. Pharmacol Exp Ther. Apr2003; 305(1):197-204.

3 Bikadi Z, Harai I, Malik D. Predicting P-gp mediated drug transport based on support vector mechanism. PLoSone. 2011:6(10):e 25815.

4 Avanti A, Kulhare P, Singh G, et al. Comparison of the efficacy and safety of moclobemide and imipramine in the treatment of depression in Indian patients. India J of Psychiatry. 2005 47(2) 84-88.

5 Preskon SH, Irwin HA. Toxicity of TCA: kinetics, mechanism, intervention. J Clin Psychiatry 1982:43:151-156.

6 Bock J, Nelson JC, Gray S et al. Desipramine hydroxylation: variability and effect of antidepressant drugs. Clin Pharmacol Ther , 1983, 33: 190-197.

7 Frank E, Kupfer DJ, Perel JM, et al. Three – years outcome for maintenance therapies in recurrent depression. Arch Gen Psychiatry, 1990, 47:1093-1099.

14

Milnacipran

Brand names:

- Toledomin
- Savella
- Ixel
- Dalcipran

Milnacipran mode of action

1. **Milnacipran is a Serotonin Re-uptake Transporter (SERT) Antagonist:** The inhibition of the serotonin reuptake pumps (SERT), located on the presynaptic neurons, by milnacipran results in increased serotonin synaptic levels.

2. **Milnacipran is a Norepinephrine Reuptake Transporter (NET) Antagonist.** The inhibition of the norepinephrine reuptake transporter (NET), located on the presynaptic norepinephrine neurons, by milnacipran results in increased synaptic norepinephrine. It appears that the inhibition of the pre synaptic NET by milnacipran is **3 times stronger** than the inhibition of SERT.

3. **Milnacipran increases dopamine levels in the prefrontal cortex by inhibition of the prefrontal NET.**
    Milnacipran's ability to block the frontal cortex norepinephrine reuptake transporters results in the increase in the prefrontal cortex dopamine levels.

4. **Milnacipran has minimal effects on H1, α1, D1, D2 and anticholinergic muscarinic receptors.** The low inhibitory effects of milnacipran on the H1, α1, D1, D2 and

anticholinergic muscarinic receptors result in a significantly lower side effect profile.

5. **At higher doses, milnacipran antagonises the NMDA receptors:**

Milnacipran NMDA antagonistic effects may be responsible for its beneficial effects on chronic pain and fibromyalgia.

The selective effects of milnacipran on the anticholinergic, histaminergic and α adrenergic receptor are summarized as follows:

- ✓ **Anticholinergic Ach muscarinic affinity: Low.** Milnacipran has a low incidence of side effects of dry mouth, constipation, blurred vision and drowsiness.
- ✓ **Histaminergic H1 affinity: Low.** Milnacipran has a low incidence of side effects of sedation and weight gain.
- ✓ **α 1 adrenergic affinity: Low.** Milnacipran has a low incidence of side effects of hypotension, dizziness, drowsiness and other cardiovascular effects.

Milnacipran has no affinity for the K^+, Na^+, Cl^- and Ca^{++} channels

Pharmacokinetics of milnacipran

Milnacipran has **linear pharmacokinetics**. Thus, any dose change leads to a proportionate change in the drug plasma levels. Thus, the higher the daily dose of milnacipran, the higher the plasma levels will get.

Milnacipran Peak plasma levels (t max): 2 hours.

Milnacipran Bioavailability: 85%

Steady State: Daily doses of milnacipran will lead to steady plasma levels within 36–48hours, which results in a significant reduction in its side effect's.

Absorption: 85%- 90%. Milnacipran is well absorbed by the gastrointestinal system, and it is not affected by the presence of food. After oral administration, milnacipran Cmax is reached within 2-4 hours.

Protein Binding: 13%. Milnacipran has *low protein binding* abilities. Only 13% of the circulating milnacipran is attached to plasma protein, while the majority of milnacipran circulates freely in the plasma.

Milnacipran Half-life (t ½): 8 hours. Milnacipran's short half-life requires a twice-a-day dosing. Moreover, due to its relatively short half-life and the lack of active metabolites, the sudden discontinuation of milnacipran may be associated with discontinuation symptoms.

Metabolism: Milnacipran is primarily metabolized by the liver via the enzyme CYP450 system **3A4** through a process of N-dealkylation. The biotransformation rate of milnacipran by the hepatic CYP 3A4 is low, indicating a low potential for drug interaction. Due to its low metabolism by the liver, no dose adjustment is needed in patients with mild liver impairment. However, milnacipran is not recommended for use in patients with chronic and severe liver failure. Furthermore, milnacipran's low hepatic metabolism allows its use in alcoholics who have no severe liver damage.

Early studies with milnacipran showed that after a single dose, the t 1/2 of milnacipran appears to be similar in healthy subjects and in subjects with mild to moderate liver impairment. However, subjects with severe hepatic impairment showed a 55% increase in t 1/2 when compared to healthy counterparts.

Elderly patients aged >65 years, require no dose adjustment as a study has shown their Cmax increases only by 30%, with the exception being if they have severely impaired renal functions. Similarly, the Cmax of milnacipran increased only by 20% in females, thus there is no need for a milnacipran dose adjustment in females.

P-gp system

The effects of milnacipran on the P-gp system are unknown.

Elimination: > 90% Urine, 10% faeces.

55% of the milnacipran dose is excreted in the urine unchanged, while 17% of milnacipran is excreted in the urine as *l-milnacipran carbamoyl-o-glucuronide*, and 8% of milnacipran is excreted in the urine as *N-desethyl milnacipran*.

Only a small fraction of milnacipran is eliminated by the faeces. In patients with renal impairment, the terminal elimination half - life of milnacipran is increased by 38% in mild renal impairment, 41% in moderate renal impairment and 122% in severe renal impairment. Thus, patients with mild renal impairment require no dose adjustment of milnacipran, while patients with moderate to severe renal dysfunction require lower doses and closer supervision.

How supplied

- Capsule   25mg, 50mg, 100mg

Dose range

- 100 mg – 200 mg for depression in divided doses
- 200mg for fibromyalgia in divided doses.

Milnacipran clinical indications

- Major depression

- Fibromyalgia
- Chronic muscular pain

Major Depressive Disorder (MDD)

Several studies have established the superiority of milnacipran over placebo in the treatment of major depression.

Patients treated with milnacipran 50mg twice a day and 100mg twice a day showed a significant improvement in their depressive symptoms and had a significantly better response compared to those patients' who got placebo.

Comparative studies of milnacipran with TCAs and SSRIs show equal efficacy (1). The long term efficacy of milnacipran has not been clearly demonstrated, and was comparable to that of placebo with regard to its ability to prevent recurrence (4). There is no evidence that milnacipran has a faster onset of action or better efficacy than other available antidepressants.

Figure 14.1 display two comparative studies of milnacipran response and remission rates versus imipramine and fluoxetine in the treatment of MDD.

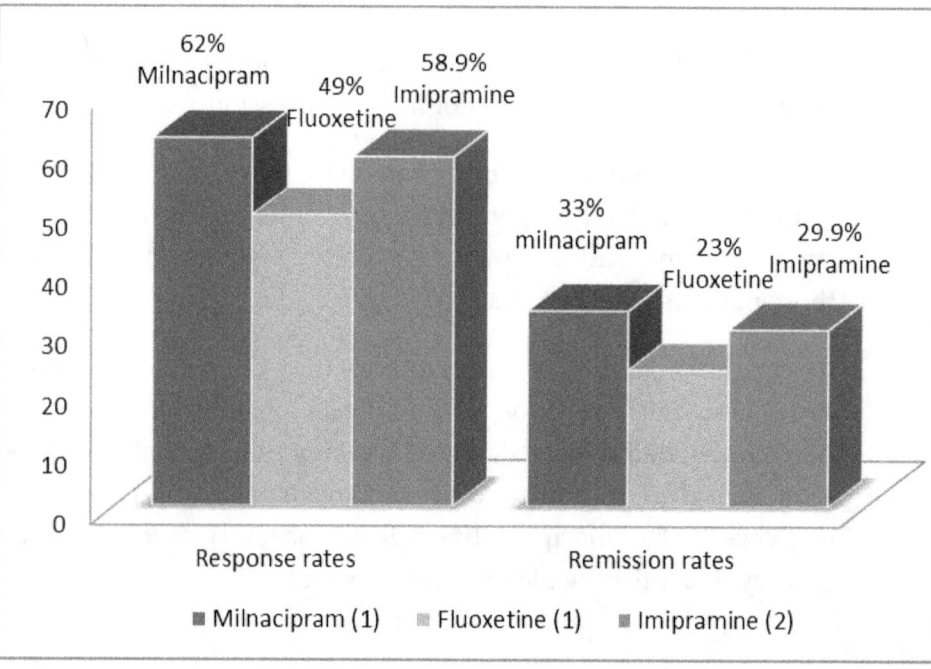

Figure 14.1: *1* **Comparative study of tha response and the remission rates of milnacipran and Fluoxetine in the treatment of MDD.** Adapted from 1. Ansseau, A., Pat P., Troisfotains B. Controlled Comparrison of milnacipran and fluoxetine in MDD. Psych. 1994:114:131-137. **2 Comparative study of milnacipran remission and response rates versus imipramine in the treatment of MDD.** Adapted from 2. Kasper S, Pletan Y, Solles A et al. Comparative studies with milnacipran and TCA in the treatment of patients with MDD. A summery of clinical trials. Int. Cl. Psych. 1996:11 (Supp. 4): 35-39.

Fibromyalgia (FM)

Fibromyalgia is a chronic condition which causes pain, stiffness, and muscle and joint tenderness.

FM also causes irritability, tiredness, chronic fatigue, mood changes, including anxiety, depression and irritability and finally sleep changes.

FM is not an arthritic-related condition since it does not cause inflammation of the joints or the muscle. The term fibromyalgia derives from the Latin word "fibro" for fibrous tissue, and from the Greek words "myo" for muscle and "algia" for pain. 80% of the patients affected with FM are predominantly women between the ages 35-55.

The causes of FM are unknown. However, studies with FM patients showed elevated spinal cord fluid levels, of substance P and nerve growth factors as well as reduced levels of the serotonin metabolite 5-HTAA. In addition, patients with FM display impaired non–REM sleep, which might explain the early-morning fatigue which is a very common symptom in patients with FM. In most cases of FM, disease onset occurs after the individual is going through a traumatic life event or infection. In other cases, FM develops in an individual who experiences high levels of stress.

The pain associated with FM is widely spread all over the body. However, it is more commonly experienced in the neck, shoulders, arms, chest and buttocks. The pain often gets worse during the period of emotional distress and during weather changes. Fatigue and muscle pain is presents in 90% of FM cases. The mental symptoms which are present in 50% of patients with FM include poor concentration, forgetfulness, irritability, anxiety and depression.

FM is also associated with body areas called "tender points" that are tender to touch. The tender points are commonly situated on the knees, the elbows, the shoulders, the hips and the back of the head. Tension headache, migraine, numbness of body areas, abdominal pain, irritable bladder and painful urination are also present in most cases of FM.

According to the Rheumatology association, the muscle pain which is associated with FM must be present longer than 3 months, and must not be accompanied by tissue swelling or inflammation.

There are several other medical conditions that may mimic FM, which include hypothyroidism, hypocalcemia, parathyroid disease, Vitamin D deficiency, polymyositis, AIDS, hepatitis, Epstein-Barr's virus and chronic depression.

It appears that the ability of milnacipran to block the serotonin and the norepinephrine reuptake transporters may be responsible for its favourable clinical effects on pain and on the other symptoms of fibromyalgia. Furthermore, it appears that the onset of its action on pain, and on the other fibromyalgia-related symptoms is much quicker than its onset of action on the mental-related symptoms.

In a double blind placebo-controlled study (5) conducted with 1025 patients diagnosed as having fibromyalgia, the patients were randomized into two groups. In one group, the patients were placed on 100mg milnacipran/day, while in the other group the patients were placed on placebo. The study was conducted over a period of 12 weeks, and it showed that the milnacipran-treated patients had significant clinical improvement compared to the placebo group, as measured by the FM Impact Questionnaire, Brief Pain Inventory (BPI) and on the Multidimensional Fatigue

Inventory total score.

Figure 14.2 shows the results of the study of milnacipran versus placebo in FM.

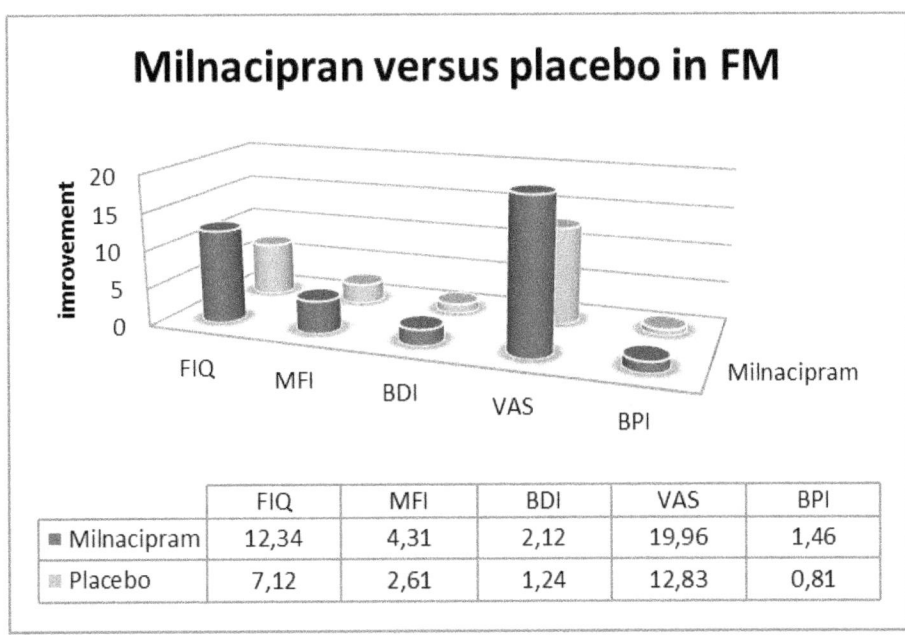

Figure 14.2.: A comparative study of 100mg/day of milnacipran versus placebo in the treatment of patients with Fibromyalgia. (Lesely M et al 2010). **FIQ**= fibromyalgia impact questionnaire, **MFI**= Multidimensional fatigue inventory, **BDI**= Beck depression inventory, **VAS**= visual analog pain score scale, **BPI**= Brief pain inventory.

How to treat with milnacipran

For major depression (MDD): start with 25 mg twice a day to be increased up to a maximum of 200mg a day.

For fibromyalgia and neuropathic pain: start with 25 mg twice a day to be increased gradually up to a maximum of 200 mg a day. Doses above 200mg were not associated with a better efficacy.

When and how to take medication

Milnacipran should be taken in two divided doses. Patients must avoid crushing or chewing the capsule as it will interfere with the drug absorption.

How to stop milnacipran

Due to its relativly short half-life, there is a need for a slow tapering of milnacipran in order to avoid withdrawal symptoms. In the event of the patient getting withdrawal symptoms, re-instate the previous dose, and once the symptoms disappear, reduce the milnacipran dose in lower proportions and over a longer period of time.

How long it takes to get an antidepressant effect

In order to get an antidepressant effect, milnacipran should be used daily for at least 2 – 4 weeks. Studies did not show increased efficacy above 200 mg a day.

Side effects of milnacipran

Most side effects of milnacipran are probably related to its ability to increase serotonin and norepinephrine in the brain. The side effects develop soon after the initiation of treatment and often disappear with time. The most common side effects of milnacipran include nausea, dry mouth, headache, sedation, weight gain, sexual dysfunction and dysuria.

Nervous system: The activation syndrome is less common for milnacipran. Common neurological side effects include:

- Insomnia
- Restlessness,
- Restless leg syndrome,
- Muscle spasm
- Tremor
- Hot flashes
- Headache
- Dizziness
- Seizures (rare, mainly associated with treatment discontinuation)
- Increased sweating
- Fatigue
- Somnolence
- Rash

Gastro-intestinal

The GI symptoms are quite common with milnacipran and usually develop within 30 minutes of drug ingestion. The GI side effects are more likely the result of the direct effect of milnacipran on the intestinal mucosa tather than the plasma peak level. The most common GI side effects of milnacipran include:

- Decreased appetite
- Nausea
- Vomiting
- Dry mouth
- Diarrhea
- Constipation
- Possible weight loss
- Gastritis 1%
- Blood in the stools

Anticholinergic
- Dry mouth
- Constipation
- Narrow angle glaucoma
- Dysuria
- Urinary retention
- Urinary hesitancy

Sexual

The sexual side effects of milnacipran are substantial and probably related to its effects on the serotonin levels. They include:

- Decreased sex drive
- Testicular pain
- Testicular swelling
- Delayed ejaculation
- Impotence
- Abnormal orgasm
- Hematuria

Suicide

The FDA requires all antidepressants to carry a black box warning stating that antidepressant may increase the risk for suicide in persons under the age of 25 years. This warning is based on data suggesting that suicidal ideations and behavior have a 2-fold increase in children and in adolescents, and a 1.5 – fold increase in the 18 – 24 age group.

Milnacipran side effects that need immediate attention

- Confusion
- Excitation
- Onset of seizure

- Yellow skin / eyes
- Severe allergic reaction
- Irregular heart beats
- Hypertension
- Induction of manic or hypomanic episode
- Activation of suicidal ideation and behaviour

Milnacipran abuse and dependence

In animal studies, milnacipran did not show abuse potential. Furthermore, in human clinical trials, there was no indication of drug seeking behaviour. However, milnacipran produces physical dependence, as evidenced by the presence of withdrawal symptoms upon abrupt discontinuation of the drug. This physical dependence on milnacipran is similar to other SNRI and SSRI drugs. However, clinicians should carefully monitor patients for signs of misuse or abuse.

Milnacipran discontinuation reaction

The sudden discontinuation of milnacipran can be associated with a discontinuation reaction, which is self-limiting. The most common symptoms of the milnacipran discontinuation reaction are:

- Irritability
- Agitation
- Dizziness
- Electric shock sensations
- Anxiety
- Confusion
- Headache
- Lethargy
- Insomnia
- Seizures

- Dysphoric mood

A slow down-titration of milnacipran is often associated with a lower risk of having the discontinuation reaction.

Safety profile of milnacipran

Use in pregnancy: FDA risk category C

Milnacipran is not evidently teratogenic.

One year of administration of milnacipran to rats did not show any hepatic changes, while two years of administration of milnacipran to rats was associated with the histologic finding of centrilobular vacuolation in male rats liver's without any liver enzymatic changes. The risk of pregnant mothers with a history of depression to develop depression during their pregnancy and especially after child delivery is very high and often requires the continuation of the treatment with SSRIs during and after the pregnancy.

The use of milnacipran during the first trimester as well as throughout the pregnancy is not recommended. Newborn children exposed to milnacipran in the maternal third trimester may develop respiratory distress, cyanosis, apnea, vomiting, hypoglycemia, hypotonia, hypertonia, tremor, jitteriness, irritability and continueous crying spells as well as feeding difficulties, temperature instability and seizures. These symptoms may result in prolonged hospitalization and may require respiratory support and tube feeding.

Use during lactation

Milnacipran is secreted in the breast milk. The maximum estimated daily infant dose of milnacipran from the breast milk was 5% of that of the maternal dose. The peak plasma concentration of milnacipran in breast milk was within 4 hours after a maternal dose. Due to its unknown effects on the newborn's normal growth and development, breast feeding should be avoided.

Milnacipran drug interactions

Milnacipran drug interaction are due to its metabolism by the liver enzyme CYP 450: 3A4.

Follows a list of milnacipran drug interactions with possible clinical consequences.

- **Warfarin:** The concomitant use May displace warfarin from its protein. This effect may increase INR, which might lead to a possible risk of bleeding.
- **Carbamazepine:** The concomitant use may cause 20% decrease in milnacipran plasma levels.
- **MAOI:** The concomitant use may cause CNS toxicity-serotonin syndrome. Patients must wait 21 days after MAOI was stopped before initiating treatment with milnacipran, while patients must wait 7 days to start MAOI after discontinuing milnacipran.
- **Epinephrine:** The concomitant use may cause hypertensive crisis and possible cardiac arrhythmia.
- **Clonidine:** The concomitant use may interfere with clonidine's antihypertensive action.
- **Tramadol:** The concomitant use may Increased risk of developing seizures.
- **Triptans:** The concomitant use may cause serotonin syndrome.

Warnings for milnacipran

> **Breast Feeding:** Try to avoid the use during pregnancy or breastfeeding: assessment of the risks versus benefits must be discussed with the patient.

- **Kidney failure**: Milnacipran should be used cautiously in patients with kidney failure.
- **Narrow-angle glaucoma**: Milnacipran use is associated with an increased risk of mydriasis due to its ability to potentiate the effects of norepinephrine (NE). Milnacipran should be avoided in patients with uncontrolled narrow-angle glaucoma.
- **Hypertension**: The effects of Milnacipran on the norepinephrine (NE) system can lead to increased heart rates and blood pressure. Milnacipran was associated with a pulse elevated by 7 beats / minute. However, further dose increases were not associated with additional increased pulse rates. Heart rate should be measured in all patients with pre-existing tachyarrhythmias.
- **ECG**: Milnacipran has no clinical effects on the ECG profiles or on the QTc interval, and it shown to be safe in the treatment of depression in patients with a history of myocardial infarction and angina.
- **Urinary hesitancy**: Milnacipran's ability to potentiate norepinephrine (NE) can increase urethral resistance, which might lead to urinary hesitancy. Male patients with dysuria, benign prostatic hyperplasia and prostatitis may be at higher risk for this side effect.
- **Testicular pain**: Milnacipran was associated with testicular pain and male ejaculation disorders.
- **Seizures**: Although milnacipran use was not associated with increased frequency of seizures, it should be given with care to patients with a history of seizures.
- **Jaundice**: Milnacipran must be discontinued in patients who develop jaundice.
- **Hyponatremia**: Milnacipran use may be associated with hyponatremia, and it is more common in the elderly and in patients taking diuretics. The symptoms of hyponatremia include headache, weakness, reduced concentration, and

confusion. In severe cases, hyponatremia can be associated with syncope, hallucinations, seizures and respiratory arrest.
- ➢ **Bleeding**: Milnacipran may increase the risk of bleeding events. Thus the concomitant use of aspirin, non steroidal anti-inflammatory medications and warfarin may increase this risk.
- ➢ **Activation of hypo -mania or mania**: Milnacipran use was associated with mania and hypomania. Milnacipran should be used cautiously in manic patients.
- ➢ **Discontinuation syndrome**: Discontinuation symptoms have been observed in patients who abruptly stopped the use of milnacipran. The most common discontinuation symptoms were dysphoric mood, agitation, sensory disturbances such as paresthesias, electric shock sensations, anxiety, irritability, headache, lethargy, insomnia and seizures. Although the discontinuation symptoms are transient and self-limiting, a gradual dose reduction of milnacipran is strongly recommended.
- ➢ **Benign prostatic hyperplasia (BPH)**: Milnacipran should be used with caution in patients with BPH due to possible urinary hesitancy and urinary retention.
- ➢ **Liver insufficiency**: Milnacipran must be avoided in patients with liver insufficiency.
- ➢ **Alcohol abuse**: Milnacipran is not recommended in patients abusing alcohol
- ➢ **MAOI**: Milnacipran requires a 2-week washout period before starting with MAOI. A 3-week washout period is required after MAOI was stopped before starting milnacipran.

Milnacipran overdose

Milnacipran **appears to be safe and not lethal in mono therapy overdose**. In clinical trials ingestion of 1000mg of milnacipran, alone or in combination with other drugs, was associated with no fatalities. However, there is a rare incidence of fatalities with milnacipran especially when milnacipran was ingested with alcohol and/ or with other central nervous depressants such as painkillers or benzo- diazepines which might cause respiratory depression.

General Symptoms of milnacipran overdose

Initially, the patient might feel extremely tired and lethargic. The pulse will slow down, and the breathing frequency will also decrease.

As the level of intoxication increases, the level of consciousness will decrease, and the patient will become unresponsive to external stimulations. The reflexes will disappear, and the breathing will get shallow. The patient's pulse and blood pressure will drop until cardiovascular system collapse.

The symptoms of milnacipran over dose are

- vomiting
- over sedation/ agitation
- dilated pupils
- abnormal heart rhythm- tachycardia
- hypertension
- cardio respiratory arrest
- confusional state
- dizziness
- increased hepatic enzymes.

What to do in case of milnacipran overdose

In general, there is no antidote for milnacipran overdose. Management is mainly supportive, aimed at maintaining respiration, pulse and blood pressure.

In the event of a recent overdose with milnacipran a stomach washout with activated charcoal might help in the elimination of the un-absorbed drug and is done with a large bore oro-gastric tube with appropriate airway protection. The aim of the stomach lavage is to get rid of the drug leftovers.

In some ER departments, ipecac is also used in order to induce vomiting of the ingested toxin, however **induction of emesis is not recommended in semi-comatose and comatose patients**. Due to the large volume of distribution of milnacipran, forced diuresis, dialysis hemo-perfusion and exchange transfusion are unlikely to be effective. Keeping open the patient's airway is compulsory, especially in semi - comatose individuals. The patient should be placed on his side in order to prevent aspiration of the vomitus back to the lungs. Suffocation due to vomit is the leading cause of death in milnacipran overdose. Blood pressure and heart rate monitoring is very important. Fluid intake should be monitored with intra -venous infusion of saline and urinary output should be also carefully monitored. In most cases, milnacipran overdose, requires hospitalization of the patient for at least 24 hours for intense observation.

Milnacipram references

1 Kasper S, Pletan Y, Solles A et al. Comparative studies with milnacipran and TCA in the treatment of patients with MDD. A summery of clinical trials. Int. Cl. Psych. 1996:11 (Supp. 4): 35-39.

2 Ansseau, A., Ppat P., Troisfotains B. Controlled Comparrison of milnacipran and fluoxetine in MDD. Psych. 1994:114:131-137.

3 Papakostas G.L, Fava M. A meta- analysis of clinical trials comparing milnacipran, an SNRI, with SSRI for the treatment of MDD. European neuropsychopharmacology, 2007: 20(17), 32 – 36.

4 Rouillon F, Warner B, Pezous N et al. Milnacipran recurrence prevention study group: milnacipram efficacy in the prevention of recurrent depression: a 12-month placebo-controlled study. Int. Clin. Psychopharmacology 2000;15:133-140.

15

Mirtazapine

Brand name: Remeron

Mode of action of mirtazapine

1. Mirtazapine is an α-2 adrenergic auto-receptor antagonist:
The inhibition of the α-2 adrenergic auto receptor results in increased release of norepinephrine and serotonin from the pre-synaptic nerve cells.

2. 5-HT2A antagonist. The 5-HT2A receptors contain 471 amino acids and are widely distributed in the central nervous system and in peripheral tissues. The inhibition of the 5-HT2A receptors situated on the GABAergic interneurons, by mirtazapine results in increased cortical dopamine.

3. 5-HT2c antagonist. The inhibition of the 5-HT2C receptors, situated on the GABAergic interneurons regulates the release of DA and NE from the prefrontal cortex.

4. 5-HT3 antagonist: The 5-HT3 receptors are located on the central and peripheral neurons. Secondary to the opening of non-selective ligand-gated channels, they produce a rapid depolarization of the cell due to a transient inward current resulting in the influx of Na+, Ca+ and the efflux of K+.

It appears that the 5-HT3 receptors are made of two subunits, namely 5-HT3a and 5-HT3b. The heterometric combination of both subunits is necessary to provide the receptor action on the cation channels. **The inhibition of the 5-HT3 receptors may be involved in cognitive enhancement as well as in nausea reduction and improved GI functions.**

The selective effects of Mirtazapine on the anticholinergic, histaminergic and α adrenergic receptors are summarized as follows:

- ✓ **Anticholinergic Ach muscarinic affinity: Low.** Mirtazapine has a low incidence of side effects of dry mouth, constipation, blurred vision and drowsiness.

- ✓ **Histaminergic H1 affinity: High.** Mirtazapine has a high incidence of side effects of sedation and weight gain.

- ✓ **α 1 adrenergic affinity: Low.** Mirtazapine has a low incidence of side effects of hypotension, dizziness, drowsiness and other cardiovascular effects.

Mirtazapine pharmacokinetics

Mirtazapine has **linear pharmacokinetics.** Thus increased doses of mirtazapine result in proportionally increased blood levels.

Absorption: Mirtazapine is well absorbed by the gastrointestinal system and **it is not affected by the presence of food in the stomach.**

Peak plasma levels (Tmax): 2 hours. The side effects of mirtazapine are dose related and tend to emerge at the peak of its plasma level. A single dosing of mirtazapine may result in emerging side effects within 2 hours after drug ingestion.

Mirtazapine Half- life (t ½): 20 – 40 hours.

Steady state: Mirtazapine reaches steady plasma levels within **5 – 7 days** of regular use.

Bioavailability 50%

Protein bounding: 85%. Mirtazapine is highly protein bound.

More than 85% of the circulating mirtazapine is attached to the plasma protein- mainly albumin.

Metabolism: 2D6, 1A2, 3A3/4. Mirtazapine is primarily metabolized by the liver by three CYP enzymes: CYP450: **2D6, 1A2** and **3A3/4.** All three liver enzymes mediate equal biotransformation of mirtazapine. The major biotransformation of mirtazapine is demethylation and hydroxylation followed by conjugation with glucuronide. In fact, 25% of mirtazapine is eliminated by the urine, conjugation with glucuronic acid.

Mirtazapine is metabolized to *desmethyl active metabolites.* However, due to their low plasma concentrations, these active metabolites have marginal clinical effects. In addition, due to its relatively short half-life and the lack of therapeutic effect of its inactive metabolites, an abrupt cessation of mirtazapine may cause severe discontinuation symptoms.

The P-gp system

Mirtazapine is not significantly affected by the P-gp system (3).

Elimination: Urine 75%, Faeces 15%. Mirtazapine is eliminated mainly by the urine. The clearance of mirtazapine can be reduced by 30% – 50% in patients with renal impairment. Thus, patients with renal impairment need to use mirtazapine cautiously due to possible drug accumulation. Elderly patients >65years may have higher blood concentration of mirtazapine as well as longer elimination half-lifes compared to young patients. In addition, female patients have been shown to have a significantly longer elimination half-life and significantly higher plasma levels of mirtazapine.

Dose range

- 15 – 45 mg once daily at bedtime for the treatment of major depression.

How supplied

- Tablets 15mg, 30mg, 45mg.
- Disintegrating tablets called Soltab15,30,45mg which dissolve on the tongue within 30 seconds

Mirtazapine clinical indications

- Major depression
- Panic disorder
- Generalized anxiety disorder (GAD)
- Post Traumatic Stress Disorder (PTSD)

Major Depressive Disorder (MDD)

In the treatment of depression mirtazapine was shown to have comparable efficacy to that of other antidepressants. The therapeutic antidepressant effects of mirtazapine can be seen after 7 – 28 days.

However, some evidence showed that mirtazapine has a somewhat faster onset of action than the SSRIs, although this faster response to mirtazapine levels out after 6 weeks of treatment. Several U.S studies have found that mirtazapine response rates were 50% as measured with the HAMD score, as compared to only a 20% response for placebo (6).

In addition, patients who poorly responded to SSRI monotherapy and were given a combination of SSRI with mirtazapine showed an additional 45% improvement compared to a 13% improvement in those who were given a combination of SSRI and placebo (7).

Another in-patient study compared the efficacy of mirtazapine and venlafaxine for a period of 8 weeks in hospitalized severely depressed patients with melancholic features. This study showed remission rates of 40% for mirtazapine and 30% for venlafaxine (8).

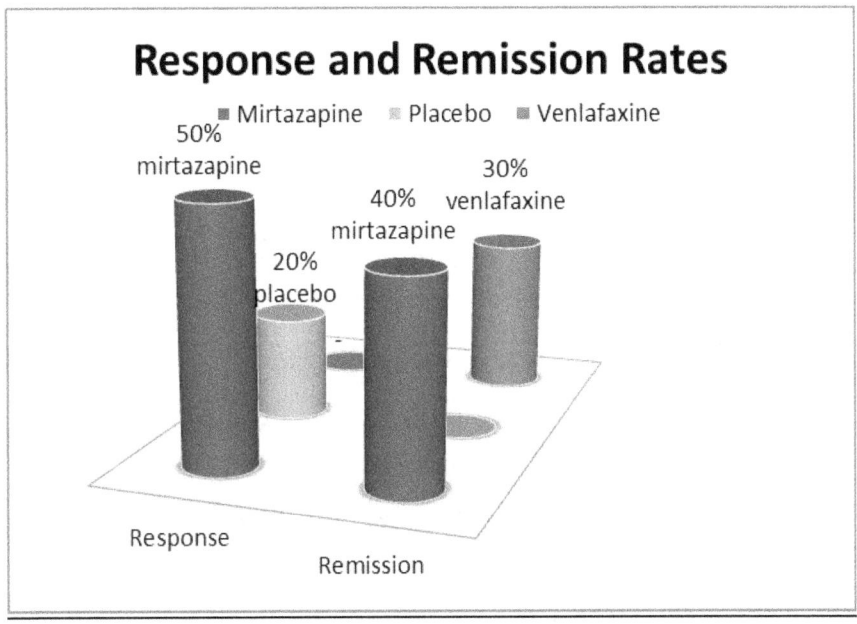

Figure 15.1 A. Response rate of mirtazapine and placebo: Adapted from Fawcett J, Barkin RL. Review of the results from clinical studies on the efficacy, safety and tolerability of mirtazapine for the treatment of patients with MDD. J Affective Disorder 1998;51:267-285. B. Remission rates of mirtazapine and venlafaxine: Adapted from Guelfi JD, Ansseau M, Timmerman L et al. Mirtazapine versus venlafaxine in hospitalized severely depressed patients with melancholic features. J Clin Psychopharmacol 2001:21:425-431.

PTSD

Mirtazapine was shown to be effective in reducing symptoms of PTSD in 50% of patients.

Oncology

Mirtazapine was shown to be a safe and effective adjunct to patients getting chemotherapy by improving nausea, anorexia, weight loss and insomnia in cancer patients.

Anxiety

Mirtazapine has shown promising results in reducing anxiety symptoms within the first week of treatment.

How to treat with mirtazapine

For depression: start with mirtazapine 15mg at bedtime and increase the dose every 7 days until you reach the desired antidepressant effect. In severe cases, a maximum of 45mg can be given once daily at bedtime.

When and how to take medication

Preferably take mirtazapine at bedtime as a-once-a-day dose.

Do not break or chew the medication as it might interfere with the drug pharmacokinetics.

How to stop mirtazapine

A sudden discontinuation of mirtazapine use can lead to discontinuation syndrome. A slow tapering of mirtazapine is recommended.

In the case of the patient getting discontinuation symptoms, re-instate the previous dose of mirtazapine, and once the symptoms disappear start reducing mirtazapine dose in a smaller proportions and over longer period of time.

How long it takes to get an antidepressant effect

In order to get an antidepressant effect, mirtazapine should be used daily for at least 2 – 4 weeks. Like all antidepressants, mirtazapine needs time before a substantial mood improvement emerges.

Side effects of mirtazapine

Most of mirtazapine's side effects develop at the beginning of treatment and usually subside with time. The most troubling side effects of mirtazapine are over-sedation and weight gain, which is probably mediated by mirtazapine's activity at the H1 histamine receptor. The most common side effects of mirtazapine are as follows:

Nervous system

- Sedation- May develop in 30% of patients
- Fatigue
- Insomnia
- Agitation
- Restlessness,
- Muscle pain
- Vivid dreams
- hallucinations
- Headache
- Dizziness
- *Seizures* (very rare)
- Rash
- Dry mouth
- Blurred vision
- Hypotension
- Palpitation

- Vertigo
- Pupil dilatation

Gastro intestinal

GI side effects are less common with mirtazapine. However, increased appetite and weight gain are highly frequent with mirtazapine use.

- *increased appetite*
- **Weight gain** – May develop in 17% of patients
- Nausea ,
- Vomiting
- Dry mouth
- Constipation

Sexual: In general, the use of mirtazapinee is associated with lower incidence of sexual dysfunction. The most common sexual side effects of mirtazapine are:

- Decreased sex drive
- Delayed ejaculation
- Impotence
- Abnormal orgasm

Other side effects
- Urinary retention
- Increased body temperature
- Excessive sweating
- Bone marrow suppression- rare
- Agranulocytosis- rare

Suicide

The FDA requires all antidepressants to carry a black box warning stating that antidepressants may increase the risk for suicide in persons under the age of 25 years. This warning is based on data suggesting that suicidal ideations and behavior has a 2 fold increase in children and in adolescents, and 1.5 – fold increase in the 18 – 24 age group.

Mirtazapine side effects that need immediate attention

- Confusion
- Excitation
- Onset of seizure
- Yellow skin / eyes
- Severe allergic reaction
- Irregular heart beats
- Hypertension/ hypotension
- Induction of manic or hypomanic episode
- Activation of suicidal ideation and behaviour

Physical & psychological dependence

Mirtazapine did not show any tendencies for drug seeking behaviours. However, patients with a history of drug abuse should be closely monitored for signs of mirtazapine misuse or abuse, which includes drug seeking behavior, development of tolerance and dose self-adjustments.

Mirtazapine discontinuation reaction

A sudden discontinuation of mirtazapine can be associated with a discontinuation reaction, the symptoms of which are self-limiting. The most common symptoms of discontinuation reaction are:

- Anxiety
- Irritability
- Agitation
- Dizziness
- Flu like symptoms

- Confusion
- Headache
- Lethargy
- Insomnia
- Seizures
- Dysphoric mood

A slow down titration of mirtazapine often reduces the risk of having the discontinuation reaction.

Safety profile of mirtazapine

Use in pregnancy: Risk category C

Mirtazapine is not evidently teratogenic.

However, the use of mirtazapine in the last trimester of pregnancy is associated with a higher incidence of respiratory distress and pulmonary hypertension, cyanosis, apnea, seizures, temperature instability, vomiting, hypoglycemia, hypotonia, hyperreflexia, tremor, irritability, constant crying and jitteriness, with subsequent prolonged hospitalization, tube feeding and respiratory support.

There is an increased risk of the newborn developing Persistent Pulmonary Hypertension of the newborn (PPHN) which is associated with substantial neonatal morbidity and mortality. In addition, reproductive studies in pregnant rats at doses 20 times the maximum recommended human dose (MRHD) showed no evidence of teratogen effects. Nevertheless, the use of mirtazapine during the first trimester as well as throughout the pregnancy is not recommended.

Use during lactation

Mirtazapine is secreted in the breast milk. Due to its unknown effects on the newborn's normal growth and development, breast-feeding should be avoided.

Carcinogenesis

There is no evidence of carcinogenesis, mutagenicity or impaired fertility with mirtazapine.

Treatment of mice and rats with doses of 20 times the maximum recommended human dose (MRHD) showed some increased incidence of hepatocellular adenoma and carcinoma in male mice at the highest dose range. The significance and the relevance of those results to humans are unknown.

Mirtazapine was not mutagenic and did not induce general DNA damage. In addition, fertility studies conducted on rats at doses 20 times the maximum recommended human dose did not affect mating and conception.

Treatment of rats at doses of mirtazapine 2 times the MRHD had no effect on mating performance, duration of gestation, or pregnancy.

Avoid using mirtzapine in the following cases
- In patients taking MAOI medication
- In patients with proven allergy to mirtazapine
- In patients with a history of seizure

Mirtazapine drug interaction

Mirtazapine drug interactions are due to its metabolism by the liver enzyme CYP 450: 2D6, 1A2 and 3A3/4.

Follows a list of mirtazapine drug interactions with the possible clinical consequences.

- **Carbamazepine:** The concomitant use may reduce mirtazapine plasma levels by 60% due to its enhanced metabolism via the liver enzyme CYP 3A4.
- **Fluvoxamine:** The concomitant use may Increases mirtazapine plasma levels by 4-fold due to its inhibition of mirtazapine metabolism.
- **Venlafaxine:** The concomitant use may cause serotonin syndrome.
- **Tramadol:** The concomitant use may increase the risk for seizures.
- **MAOI:** The concomitant use may cause CNS toxicity - serotonin syndrome. Wait 21 days after MAOI was stopped before initiating treatment with mirtazapine. Wait 5-7 days after discontinuing mirtazapine before starting MAOI.
- **Methylphenidate:** The concomitant use may cause mania in patients with bipolar mood disorder.
- **Fluoxetine:** The concomitant use may increase mirtazapine blood levels.

Warnings for mirtazapine

- **Pregnancy: Risk category C.** Try to avoid the use during pregnancy or breastfeeding. Assessment of the risks versus benefits must be discussed with the patient.
- **Mirtazapine may cause an increase in suicidal risk in young adults.** Pooled analysis of trials of drugs used for MDD showed that SNRIs and SSRIs may increase the risk

of suicidal thinking and behavior in children, adolescents and young adults aged 18-24. The use of **any** antidepressants in this population must balance the risk of suicide with the clinical need. Careful monitoring of the patient's clinical worsening, and suicidality should also involve the family and all other caregivers cause increases in suicidal risk in young adults.

- **Activation of hypomania or mania** occurred in 0.2% of mirtazapine treated bipolar patients. However, as mirtazapine may trigger mania in predisposed patients, it should be used cautiously in patients with a history of bipolar mood disorder
- **The incidence of seizures** is extremely low with mirtazapine use. In all the US clinical trials only one seizure was reported. However, mirtazapine should be used cautiously in patients with a history of seizures
- **Serotonin syndrome** may develop with mirtazapine use.
- **Cardiac impairment**: Mirtazapine needs to be used with caution in patients with cardiac impairment.
- **Co-administration of mirtazapine with tramadol** may increase seizure risk.
- **Renal impairment**: mirtazapine requires a dose adjustment (lower dose) in mild to moderate renal impairment.
- **Alcohol**: Mirtazapine is not recommended in patients abusing alcohol.
- **Elderly**: Mirtazapine needs a dose adjustment (lower dose) in the elderly
- **MAOI:** Mirtazapine combined with MAOI might be fatal. Mirtazapine requires a **7-day** washout period before starting with MAOI. After stopping a MAOI, a **3-week** washout period is required before starting mirtazapine.
- **Withdrawal reaction.** Mirtazapine may cause withdrawal reaction, prevention of which requires a slow reduction of

mirtazapine doses. The onset of withdrawal symptoms is attributed to mirtazapine's short half-life as well as to the lack of active metabolites. The withdrawal symptoms of mirtazapine can develop as early as the second day of the drug's sudden discontinuation and may persist for several days. The most common withdrawal symptoms are nausea, dizziness, insomnia, anxiety, tension and headache.

- **Agranulocytosis**: in clinical trials there were **three** cases of agranulocytosis out of 2796 patients treated with mirtazapine. Thus patients should be observed for signs of sore throat, fever, stomatitis or any other signs of infection, and labs should be checked for low WBC count with any signs of infection.
- **Cholesterol**: Non-fasting cholesterol increased by >20% above the upper normal limits in 15% of the patients treated with mirtazapine as compared to 7% for placebo.
- **Triglycerides:** Non-fasting triglycerides increased to >500mg/dL in 6% of patients treated by mirtazapine as compared to 3% of patients on placebo.
- **Transaminase elevation.** Treatment with mirtazapine caused clinically significant SGPT elevations >3 times the upper normal limit in 2% of patients. However, the transaminase elevation was not associated with compromised liver function.
- **Increased appetite:** weight gain developed in 17% of the patients treated with mirtazapine as compared to 2% for placebo.
- **Somnolence:** somnolence was reported in 54% of the patients treated with mirtazapine compared to 18% on placebo. Somnolence was associated with treatment discontinuation in 10% of mirtazapine treated patients. In addition, increased somnolence may affect performance in activities which require alertness.

Mirtazapine overdose

Mirtazapine overdose can be either un-intentional or intentional.

The effects of mirtazapine overdose also depend on whether it was ingested alone or as a combination with other drugs and/ or alcohol. As a general rule, the bigger the amount of mirtazapine ingested, the worse the reaction will get and the higher the possibility for lethal results.

General symptoms of mirtazapine overdose

Initially, the patient might feel extremely tired and lethargic. The pulse will slow down, and the breathing frequency will decrease. As the level of intoxication increases, the level of consciousness will decrease, and the patient will become unresponsive to external stimulations. The reflexes will disappear, and the breathing will get shallow. The patient's pulse and blood pressure will drpop until cardiovascular system collapse

Mirtazapine is **relatively safe in mono therapy overdose,** with rare incidence of fatalities. However, the concomitant use of mirtazapine with alcohol and with other central nervous depressants such as painkillers or benzo-diazepines may result in death caused by respiratory depression.

Symptoms of mirtazapine over dose are

- Over-sedation
- drowsiness
- disorientation
- impaired memory
- Seizure
- abnormal heart rhythm
- tachycardia
- hallucinations

- vomiting
- loss of consciousness

What to do in the case of overdose

In general, there is no antidote for mirtazapine overdose. Management is mainly supportive, aimed at maintaining respiration, pulse and blood pressure. In the event of a recent overdose with mirtazapine a stomach washout with activated charcoal might help in the elimination of the un-absorbed drug and is done with a large bore oro-gastric tube with appropriate airway protection. The aim of the stomach lavage is to get rid of the drug leftovers.

In some ER departments, ipecac is also used in order to induce vomiting of the ingested toxin, however **induction of emesis is not recommended in semi-comatose and comatose patients**.

Due to the large volume of distribution of mirtazapine, forced diuresis, dialysis hemo-perfusion and exchange transfusion are unlikely to be effective. Keeping open the patient's airway is compulsory, especially in semi - comatose individuals.

The patient should be placed on his side in order to prevent aspiration of the vomitus back to the lungs. Suffocation due to vomit is the leading cause of death in mirtazapine overdose.

Blood pressure and heart rate monitoring is very important. Fluid intake should be monitored with intra -venous infusion of saline and urinary output should be also carefully monitored. In most cases, mirtazapine overdose, requires hospitalization of the patient for at least 24 hours for intense observation.

Mirtazapine References

1 Akamine, Yumiko,Yasui-Furukori et al. Psychotropic drug – drug interactions involving P-gp. Nov 2012 Vol 26 issue 11- 959 – 973.

2 Weiss j, Dormann SM, Martin- Facklam et al. Inhibition of P-gp by newer antidepressants. J. Pharmacol Exp Ther. Apr 2003; 305(1):197-204.

3 Uhr M,Grauer MT, Holsboer F. Differential enhancement of antidepressant penetration into the brain in mice with abcb1ab P-gp gene disruption. Biol Psychiatry, Oct 2003; 15:54(8):840-846.

4 Szegedi A, Muller MJ, Anghelescu I Early improvement under mirtazapine and paroxetine predicts later stable response and remission with high sensitivity in patients with MDD. J of Clin Psychiatry. 2003; 64 (4):413-420.

5 Thase ME. Effectiveness of antidepressants: comparative remission rates. J Clin Psychiatry 2003: 64(Suppl 2): 3-7.

6 Fawcett J, Barkin RL. Review of the results from clinical studies on the efficacy, safety and tolerability of mirtazapine for the treatment of patients with MDD. J Affective Disorder 1998;51:267-285.

7 Carpenter LL, Yasmin S, Price L. A double blind, placebo controlled study of antidepressant augmentation with mirtazapine. Biol Psychiatry 2002;51:183-188.

8 Guelfi JD, Ansseau M, Timmerman L et al. Mirtazapine versus venlafaxine in hospitalized severely depressed patients with melancholic features. J Clin Psychopharmacol 2001:21:425-431.

9 Freund TF, Gulyas AL. Inhibitory control of GABAergic

interneurons in the hippocampus. Can J Physiol Pharmacol. 1997 May; 75(5): 479-87

10 McMahon Lori L, Kauer J.A. Hippocampal Interneurons Express a Novel Form of Synaptic Plasticity. Neouron, February 1997, Vol 18, 295-305.

16

Paroxetine

Brand names: Aropax, Paxil

Mode of action of paroxetine

1. Paroxetine is a Serotonin Reuptake Transporter (SERT) antagonist

The inhibition of the SERT located on the presynaptic neurons by paroxetine, results in increased serotonin synaptic levels. Out of all the SSRIs, paroxetine is the most potent inhibitor of the SERT (1). The occupancy of the SERT by paroxetine reaches 75 - 93% at doses of 20mg, suggesting that the 20mg starting dose of paroxetine results in the minimum 80% occupancy required to get a clinical response.

2. Paroxetine is a Norepinephrine Reuptake Transporter (NET) antagonist.

Paroxetine's inhibition of NET, located on the pre synaptic nerve cell, results in increased synaptic levels of NE. Out of all the SSRIs, paroxetine is the most potent inhibitor of the NET. However, the inhibitory property of paroxetine on the NET is much weaker than its effects on the SERT. Inhibition of the NET becomes evident only at a dose of paroxetine of 40mg a day.

3. **Nitric Oxide Synthase (NOS) enzyme inhibitor**. Paroxetine may inhibit NOS enzymes. This effect of paroxetine probably contributes, along with its effects on serotonin, to the sexual dysfunction side effects of paroxetine.

The selective effects of paroxetine on the anticholinergic, histaminergic and α adrebnergic receptors are summarized as follows:

- ✓ **Muscarinic M1 receptors affinity. Low.** Paroxetine has a mild inhibitory effect on the M1 muscarinic receptors which can lead to mild anticholinergic effects, which include dry mouth, constipation and blurred vision.

- ✓ **Histaminergic H1 receptors affinity: Low.** Paroxetine has a low incidence of side effects of sedation and weight gain.

- ✓ **α 1 adrenergic receptors affinity: Low.** Paroxetine has a low incidence of side effects of hypotension, dizziness, drowsiness and other cardiovascular effects.

Pharmacokinetics of paroxetine

Paroxetine has **non-linear pharmacokinetics,** and it *inhibits* its own metabolism. Thus, a dose increase of paroxetine may result in a disproportionate increase in paroxetine plasma levels. Therefore, the higher the daily dose of paroxetine, the greater the plasma level will get. In addition, paroxetine has a strong age-related plasma drug fluctuation.

Thus, the same dose of paroxetine can lead up to 100% higher plasma levels in individuals above 65 years of age compared to younger individuals. These age-related blood level differences may be responsible for the possible increase in side effects in those aged above 65. Paroxetine is completely absorbed after oral ingestion.

When administered with food, its Cmax is 29% greater amd its Tmax is reached at 4.9 hours rather than 6.4 hours on an empty stomach.

Peak plasma level time: (Tmax): 6.4 hours– on empty stomach. **4.9 hours** when ingested with food.

Peak plasma levels are lower in young males compared to individuals above the age of 65. In general, paroxetine side effects are usually dose related and tend to emerge when the drug reaches its peak plasma level.

Steady state: Daily ingestion of paroxetine will result in steady plasma levels within **7-10 days**.

Protein bounding: **95%**. Paroxetine is highly protein bound.

Bioavailability: 100%

Half-life (t 1/2): 21 - 24 hours. Due to its relatively short half-life and the lack of a therapeutic effect of its metabolites, abrupt cessation of paroxetine can result in a severe discontinuation syndrome. In fact, paroxetine has the worst withdrawal symptom profile amongst all the SSRIs. In addition, due to its high lipid solubility, and its small molecular size, paroxetine can readily pass through the blood – brain barrier in a very high proportion.

Metabolism: Paroxetine is primarily metabolized by the liver via the enzyme CYP450: **2D6**. Studies have shown that there are more than 80 genetic variants of the CYP 2D6 iso- enzymes. Four variants have been identified as responsible for poor metabolism of paroxetine. Patients who have this 2D6 variant that results in poor paroxetine metabolism may experience an unusually higher paroxetine blood level, which is similar to those patients who have a liver disease. Poor metabolizers and patients with compromised livers require lower doses of paroxetine to avoid excessive accumulation of the drug in the blood.

Paroxetine is metabolized into products conjugated with glucuronic acid and sulphate. These metabolites are clinically inactive.

Elimination: Urine 65%, Faeces 36%. Paroxetine is eliminated mainly by the urine and in a smaller proportion in the faeces. The elimination of paroxetine is mostly in the form of its metabolites. Only less than 1% of paroxetine is excreted unchanged. Thus, patients with renal impairment need to use paroxetine cautiously due to possible drug accumulation.

P-gp System

Paroxetine is **a potent inhibitor of the P-gp** system in vivo and in vitro (3). The inhibitory effects of paroxetine on the P-gp system might interfere with the plasma levels of other co – administered drugs which are also P-gp substrates. Furthermore, the P-gp system's presence in the blood-brain barrier may be an important factor limiting the entry of paroxetine (as well as amitriptyline, venlafaxine doxepine citalopram and trimipramine) into the brain (4).

How supplied

- Tablet: 10mg, 20mg, 30mg, 40 mg,
- Controlled released tablets (CR): 12.5mg, 25mg
- Oral solution 10mg/ 5ml

Dose range

- 20 mg – 50 mg for depression

Clinical indications

- Major depression
- Panic disorder
- Obsessive compulsive disorder
- Premenstrual dysphoric disorder
- Post Traumatic Stress Disorder
- Generalised anxiety disorder
- Social anxiety disorder

Panic disorder (PD)

Paroxetine was the first SSRI to get FDA approval for the treatment of PD. Currently, all the SSRIs are indicated for the treatment of PD. The treatment with paroxetine requires a lower starting dose of 10 mg a day in order to avoid worsening of the anxiety symptoms which are common at the initial phase of treatment. A gradual and slow dose increase can be given as clinically indicated. Although the currently available data suggest that the effective dose of paroxetine for PD is 40 mg a day, individual variation seems to suggest that some individuals may benefit from a lower dose.

The overall duration of treatment for PD with paroxetine is 6 – 12 months. However, in some cases a longer period of treatment is required with the possibility of continuing treatment indefinitely.

Major Depressive Disorder (MDD)

Several studies have established the superiority of paroxetine over placebo in the treatment of major depression. However, within the SSRI class, there is no evidence for superior effectiveness of any SSRI over another. Furthermore, it appears that there is no direct relationship between paroxetine's plasma concentration and its clinical response. Figure 15.2 shows two studies of paroxetine: the first is a response study of paroxetine versus nefazodone(5), and the second is a remission study of paroxetine versus duloxetine (6).

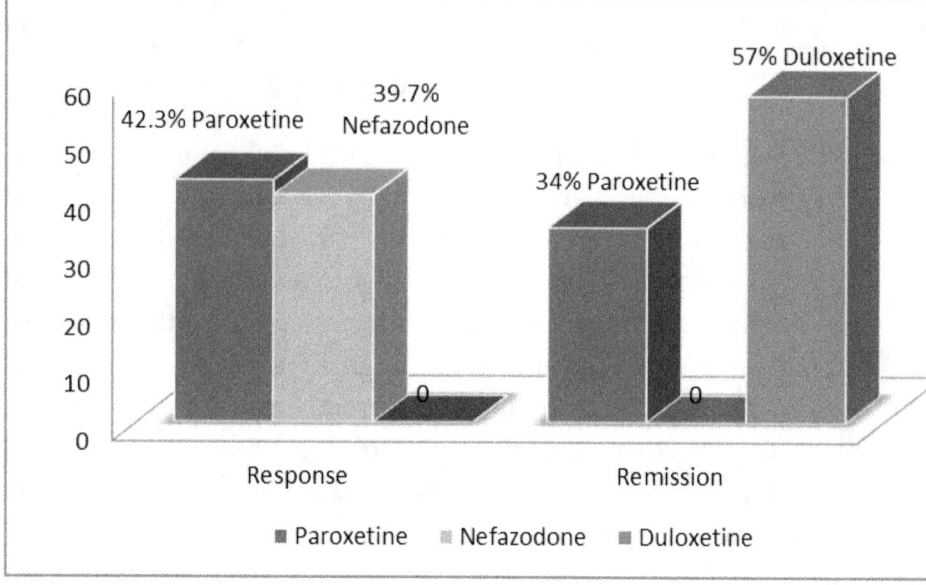

Figure 16.1: A) **Response study of paroxetine compared to nefazodone**: Adapted from Baldwin DS, Hawley CJ, Abed RT et al. A multicentre double blind comparison of nefazodone and paroxetine in the treatment of outpatients with moderate to severe depression. J Clin Psychiatry 1996;57 (2):46-52.

B) **Remission study of paroxetine compared to duloxetine**: Adapted from Goldstein DJ, Lu Y, Detka M et al. Duloxetine in the treatment of depression: a double blind placebo controlled comparison with paroxetine. J Cl Psychopharmacology August 2004; Vol 24 (4) 389 – 399.

In addition, paroxetine has been shown to have long-term efficacy. The incidence of recurrence of depression in patients receiving maintenance therapy with paroxetine was significantly lower than that of patients getting a placebo.

Only 16% of the patients treated with paroxetine relapsed, compared to 43% of those patients who got placebo (7). Another long-term study in MDD patients compared paroxetine, imipramine and placebo; a 25% relapse rates was obsereved in the placebo group, while only 15% of the patients relapsed in the paroxetine group, and 4% in the imipramine group (8).

OCD

Paroxetine, like other SSRIs, has been shown to have efficacy for the treatment of OCD, independent of the patient's mood. In general, the average dose of paroxetine for the treatment of OCD is 40mg a day, and it requires 3 to 12 weeks of treatment before a clinical improvement occurs.

Post traumatic stress disorder (PTSD)

Paroxetine was shown to be effective in the treatment of PTSD, both in the acute phase as well as for long term use.

Premenstrual Dysphoric Disorder (PMDD)

Paroxetine was shown to be effective in reducing the physical and the psychological symptoms of PMDD in doses of 20mg a day.

Social anxiety disorder

Paroxetine is effective for the treatment of Social anxiety disorder with an optimal daily dose of 20mg.

Generalised Anxiety Disorder (GAD)

Paroxetine was shown to be effective in the treatment of the acute phase of GAD, as well as for long-term use at dose levels of 20 mg – 40 mg a day.

The effects of paroxetine on the symptoms of GAD can last up to 6 months after the treatment was terminated.

How to treat

For Major Depression (MDD): For paroxetine- Start with 20mg a day in a single morning dose. Wait at least two weeks to assess the clinical improvement before increasing the dose to a maximum of 50mg a day.

For paroxetine CR, an initial dose of 25mg a day may be increased by 12.5 mg/day weekly to a maximum of 62.5mg/day.

- **For OCD:** For paroxetine Start with 20mg a day to be increased weekly by 10 mg up to 60 mg a day if necessary.

- **For Panic disorder (PD), Social anxiety & Post Traumatic Stress disorder (PTSD):** Start with 10mg a day to avoid excitation and possible anxiety, and increase the dose weekly in increments of 10mg/day to a maximum of 40mg a day. As a general rule, the higher the patient's anxiety, the *lower* the starting dose should be and the *slower* the dose increases.

- **For Premenstrual dysphoric disorder (PMDD):** Start with paroxetine CR 12.5 mg a day, initiating a week before the menses start. In severe cases take the medicine throughout the menstrual cycle at a maximum dose of 25mg a day.

When to take medication: Evening

Patients should take paroxetine preferably in the evening. However, paroxetine can be taken at any time of the day if it is tolerated.

How to stop paroxetine

Due to its short half-life and the lack of active metabolites paroxetine has a strong potential for withdrawal syndrome, which requires a slow down-titration. The patient need to reduce the dose of paroxetine gradually, with a 50% dose reduction every 3 days.

In the case of the patient experiencing withdrawal symptoms, re-instate the previous dose, and once the symptoms disappear, start reducing the paroxetine dose in a smaller proportions and over a longer period of time. In the event of patients getting severe withdrawal symptoms, the dose of paroxetine should be reduced slowly over several months. Alternatively, add another SSRI with a longer half-life (such as fluoxetine) to prevent severe withdrawal symptoms. Once fluoxetine reaches its steady state, then the patient can stop the paroxetine and remain only on the fluoxetine which then can be gradually tapered off.

How long it takes to get an antidepressant effect

In order to get an antidepressant effect, paroxetine should be used daily for at least 2 – 4 weeks.

Like all antidepressants, paroxetine requires time before a substantial mood improvement can be evident. Paroxetine's efficacy can be increasing via increasing the dose; many patients experience a beneficial effect with 50mg of paroxetine.

Side effects of paroxetine

Paroxetine's side effects are related to its ability to increase serotonin in the brain as well as in other organs. Most side effects develop soon after the initiation of treatment with paroxetine, and often disappear with time. The most common side effects of paroxetine are:

Nervous system

- Activation. The activation response is much less common for paroxetine compared to other SSRI medications
- Insomnia
- Agitation,
- Restlessness,
- Jitteriness
- Anxiety
- Tremor,
- Increased sweating
- Flushing
- Headache
- Dizziness
- Seizures (rare)
- Somnolence
- Cognitive slowing
- Reduced attention
- Apathy
- Emotional blunting
- Rash

Gastro intestinal: The GI symptoms are more common with paroxetine and usually develop within 30 minutes of the drug ingestion. They are more likely the result of the direct effect of paroxetine on the intestinal mucosa than to its plasma peak level.

- decreased appetite
- upper gastrointestinal symptoms
- nausea,
- vomiting
- dry mouth
- diarrhoea

- constipation
- possible weight loss

Sexual:

The incidence of sexual side effects attributed to the SSRIs is approximately between 20% - 40% of treated patients. The sexual side effects of paroxetine are dose-dependent and do not diminish over time. The most common sexual side effects are:

- Decreased sex drive
- Delayed ejaculation
- Impotence
- Inability to reach an orgasm

Suicide

The FDA requires all antidepressants to carry a black box warning stating that antidepressant may increase the risk of suicide in persons under the age of 25 years. This warning is based on data suggesting that suicidale ideations and behavior have a 2-fold increase in children and in adolescents, and a 1.5-fold increase in the 18 – 24 age group.

How to manage paroxetine side effects: General Practical implication

The side effects of paroxetine are often dose dependent: the higher the dose of paroxetine, the worse the side effects.. Reducing the dose of paroxetine is often associated with resolution of the side effects. See above for recommendations for appropriate paroxetine dose reductions.

Paroxetine side effects that requires immediate attention:

- Confusion
- Excitation

- Onset of seizure
- Yellow skin / eyes
- Severe allergic reaction
- Irregular heart beats
- Low blood pressure
- Bruising and bleeding(relatively rare)
- Induction of manic episode
- Activation of suicidal ideation and behaviour

Physical and psychological dependence

In animal studies, paroxetine did not show abuse potential. Furthermore, in human clinical trials, there was no evidence of drug seeking behaviour, euphoria and drug liking. However, paroxetine can cause physical dependence as evidenced by the presence of withdrawal symptoms upon abrupt discontinuation of the drug. This physical dependence on paroxetine is similar to the other SNRIs and SSRIs. In general, clinicians should carefully monitor the patients for signs of misuse or abuse.

Paroxetine discontinuation reaction

A sudden discontinuation of paroxetine may be associated with a discontinuation reaction. The discontinuation symptoms are usually self-limiting. The most common symptoms of the paroxetine discontinuation reaction are:

- nausea
- insomnia
- dizziness
- light-headedness
- vertigo
- nightmares and vivid dreams
- feelings of electricity in the body
- anxiety

Safety profile of paroxetine

Use in pregnancy: Risk category D

Epidemiological studies have shown that infants exposed to paroxetine in the first trimester of pregnancy have an increased risk of congenital malformations. The most common was cardiovascular malformations, which were observed in 2% of the paroxetine exposed infants. The specificcardiovascular malformations in the paroxetine exposed infants were ventricular septal defects (VSDs) and atrial septal defects (ASDs).

In addition, the use of paroxetine in the last trimester of pregnancy is associated with higher incidence of respiratory distress and persistent pulmonary hypertension of the newborn (PPHN) which is associated with high neonatal mortality. Neonates exposed to paroxetine late in the third trimester may develop complications soon after the delivery, which include respiratory distress, cyanosis, apnea, seizures, vomiting, hypoglycemia, hypertonia, hyperreflexia, tremor, jitteriness, constant crying, temperature instability and feeding difficulties, which may subsequently require prolonged hospitalization, respiratory support and tube feeding.

Based on the current available data, the use of paroxetine during the first trimester as well as throughout the pregnancy is not recommended, and other antidepressants should be considered.

Use during lactation

Paroxetine is secreted in the breast milk. Due to its unknown effects on the newborn's normal growth and development, breast-feeding should be avoided.

Paroxetine's drug interaction

Paroxetine's drug interactions are due to its metabolism by the liver enzymes CYP 450 2D6.

Follows a list of paroxetine's drug interactions and the possible clinical consequences.

- **Warfarin:** The concomitant use may cause a 65% increase in warfarin blood levels, which carries the risk of bleeding. In addition, paroxetine may increase INR.
- **Phenytoin:** The concomitant use may increase phenytoin blood levels.
- **MAOI:** The concomitant use may cause Serotonin syndrome. Patients need to wait at least 21 days after the MAOI was stopped before initiating treatment with paroxetine. Patient who stop paroxetine need to wait at least 7 days before they can start MAOI.
- **Benztropine & Procyclidine:** The concomitant use may increase benztropine/procyclidine plasma levels by up to 40%.
- **Lithium:** The concomitant use may increase the concomitant use may increase.
- **Pimozide & Thioridazine:** The concomitant use may increase plasma levels of both antipsychotics which can subsequently cause cardiac arrhythmias.
- **Digoxin:** The concomitant use may **decrease digoxine plasma levels by 18%.**
- **Tramadol: The concomitant use may cause serotonin syndrome.**
- **LSD:** The concomitant use may cause grand mal seizures and worsening of flashbacks.
- **Sumatryptans:** The concomitant use may cause weakness and in-coordination.

- **Cimetidine:** The concomitant use may result in 50% increase in paroxetine plasma levels.
- **Ritonavir:** The concomitant use may result in a significant decrease in paroxetine plasma levels.

Warnings for paroxetine

> **Pregnancy: Risk category D.** The use of paroxetine during pregnancy should be avoided. Assessment of the risks versus benefits needs to be discussed with the patient.
> **MAOI:** Paroxetine may cause serotonin syndrome when it is used in combination with MAOIs. Paroxetine users require at least 2 weeks of a washout period before starting with MAOI and 7 days befor switching from MAOI to paroxetine.
> **Elderly:** Paroxetine needs a dose reduction in the elderly.
> **Liver impairment:** Paroxetine needs a dose reduction in patient's with liver impairment.
> **Kidney impairment:** Paroxetine needs a dose reduction in patients with kidney impairment.
> **Activation of hypomania or mania** occurred in **1%** of paroxetine-treated patients compared to 0.3% of placebo-treated patients. In bipolar patients, the rates of manic exacerbation was 2.2% for the paroxetine-treated patients.
> **The incidence of seizures** is **0.1%** among the paroxetine-treated patients.
> **Discontinuation response** may develop when paroxetine is stopped abruptly. The most common discontinuation symptoms include dysphoric mood, agitation, anxiety, dizziness, irritability, paresthesias in the form of electric shock sensations, headaches, insomnia, emotional lability, lethargy and confusion. A gradual dose reduction is strongly recommended.
> **Hyponatremia** may develop subsequent to the use of paroxetine, especially in volume-depleted patients and in

patients on diuretics. The symptoms of hyponatremia include headaches, reduced concentration, confusion, weakness and unsteadiness, which may lead to falls. Severe cases of hyponatremia may result in seizures, hallucinations, respiratory arrest, coma and death.
- **Akathisia** was observed in paroxetine-treated patients and is characterized by an inner sense of restlessness, psychomotor agitation, and an inability to sit still. It is associated with significant distress.
- **Angle–closure glaucoma**: Paroxetine may have an effect on the pupil size resulting in mydriasis. Patients with narrow-angle glaucoma may experience increased intraocular pressure when treated with paroxetine.
- **Abnormal bleeding** was observed in patients using paroxetine. Concomitant use of warfarin, NSAIDs and aspirin may add to this risk.

Paroxetine overdose

Paroxetine is *rarely lethal in monotherapy overdose*. However, the concomitant use of paroxetine with alcohol and/ or with other central nervous depressants such as painkillers or benzodiazepines may result in death caused by respiratory depression.

General symptoms of paroxetine overdose

Initially, the patient might feel extremely tired and lethargic. The pulse will slow down, and the breathing frequency will also decrease. As the level of intoxication increases, the level of consciousness will decrease, and the patient will become unresponsive to external stimulations. The reflexes will disappear, and the breathing will get shallow. The patient's pulse and blood pressure will drop until cardiovascular system collapse.

Symptoms of paroxetine over dose include

- somnolence
- nausea
- vomiting
- over sedation
- agitation
- confusion
- dizziness
- dilated pupils (mydriasis
- abnormal heart rhythm
- tachycardia
- bradycardia
- torsades de pointes
- hypertension
- stupor
- coma
- convulsions
- status epilepticus
- dystonia
- rhabdomyolysis
- myoclonus
- urinary retention
- acute renal failure
- hepatic dysfunction

What to do in the case of overdose

In general, there is no antidote for paroxetine overdose. Management is mainly supportive, aimed at maintaining respiration, pulse and blood pressure. In the event of a recent overdose with paroxetine, a stomach-washout with activated charcoal might help in the elimination of the un-absorbed drug and is done with a large bore oro-gastric tube with appropriate airway protection. The aim of the stomach lavage is to get rid of the drug leftovers.

In some ER departments, ipecac is also used in order to induce vomiting of the ingested toxin, however **induction of emesis is not recommended in semi-comatose and comatose patients**. Due to the large volume of distribution of paroxetine, forced diuresis, dialysis hemo-perfusion and exchange transfusion are unlikely to be effective. Keeping open the patient's airway is compulsory, especially in semi - comatose individuals. The patient should be placed on his side in order to prevent aspiration of the vomitus back to the lungs. Suffocation due to vomit is the leading cause of death in paroxetine overdose. Blood pressure and heart rate monitoring is very important. Fluid intake should be monitored with intra-venous infusion of saline and urinary output should be also carefully monitored. In most cases, paroxetine overdose requires hospitalization of the patient for at least 24 hours for intense observation.

Paroxetine references

1 Hiemke C, Haarter S, et al. Pharmacokinetics of SSRI. Pharmacol Ther 2000;85:11 - 28.

2 Akamine, Yumiko, Yasui-Furukori et al. Psychotropic drug – drug interactions involving P-gp. Nov 2012 Vol 26 issue 11- 959 - 973.

3 Weiss j, Dormann SM, Martin- Facklam et al. Inhibition of P-gp by newer antidepressants. J. Pharmacol Exp Ther. Apr 2003; 305(1):197-204.

4 Jun-Sheng W, Hao-Jie Z. Bryan BG et al. Sertraline and its metabolite desmethylsertraline, but not Buproprion or its three major metabolites, have high affinity for P-gp. Biol Pharm Bull Feb 2008; 31(2): 231 - 234.

5 Baldwin DS, Hawley CJ, Abed RT et al. A multicentre double blind comparison of nefazodone and paroxetine in the treatment of outpatients with moderate to severe depression. J Clin Psychiatry 1996;57 (2):46-52.

6 Goldstein DJ, Lu Y, Detka M et al. Duloxetine in the treatment of depression: a double blind placebo controlled comparison with paroxetine. J Cl Psychopharmacology August 2004;Vol 24 (4) 389 – 399.

7 Montgomery SA, Dunbar G,. Paroxetine is better than placebo in relapse prevention and the prophylaxis of recurrent depression. Int Clin Psychopharmacology 1993;8: 189 – 195.

8 Claghorn JL, Feighner JP, et al A double blind comparison of paroxetine with imipramine in the long term treatment of depression. J Clin Psychopharmacology , 1993;13(2): 23-27.

17

Sertraline

Brand name: Zoloft

Sertraline's mode of action

1 Sertraline is a SERT antagonist: The inhibition of the SERT located on the presynaptic neurons by sertraline results in increased serotonin synaptic levels. The potency of sertraline in blocking the SERT is second only to paroxetine (3). The occupancy of the SERT by sertraline is 85% at doses of 150mg, suggesting that the starting dose of sertraline 50mg can achieve the desired clinical response.

2 Sertraline is a Dopamine Reuptake Transporter (DAT) antagonist. The inhibition of DAT results in increased synaptic dopamine levels. However, in comparison to its effects on SERT, the inhibitory effects of sertraline on the DAT are _very weak,_ less than 5% its effects on the SERT. The affinity of sertraline to the DAT is only 11% at a dose of 50-100mg.

The selective effects of sertraline on the anticholinergic, histaminergic and α adrenergic receptors are summarized as follows:

- ✓ **Muscarinic M1 receptors affinity. Low.** Sertraline has a mild inhibitory effect on the M1 muscarinic receptors which can lead to mild anticholinergic effects, which include dry mouth, constipation and blurred vision.

- ✓ **Histaminergic H1 receptors affinity: Low.** Sertraline has a low incidence of side effects of sedation and weight gain.

✓ **α 1 adrenergic receptors affinity: Moderte.** The inhibitory effect of sertraline on the α1 adrenoreceptors is 10 fold stronger than that of the other SSRIs (3). Fortunately, this high affinity for the α1 receptor does not have clinical repercussions. Thus sertraline has low incidence of side effects of hypotension, dizziness, increased heart rates and drowsiness.

Dopamine D2 receptor: The inhibition of the D2 receptors by sertraline may have some antipsychotic effects, which makes sertraline an important drug for the treatment of psychotic depression.

Sigma-1 receptor: The inhibitory effects of sertraline on the Sigma1 receptors may be involved with its anxiolytic effects.

Sertraline pharmacokinetics

Absorption: Sertraline has **linear pharmacokinetics.** Thus, any dose change leads to a proportional change in the drug plasma levels. The higher the daily dose of sertraline, the higher the plasma level will get.

Sertraline is absorbed slowly by the gastrointestinal system, and its absorption is accelerated by the presence of food. Sertraline's Cmax increases by 25% when it is taken with food, while its Tmax decreases from 8 hours to 5.5-hours. Therefore, due to this acceleration of sertraline's absorption with food, it is strongly recommended to take sertraline with meals.

Peak plasma levels (Tmax): 6 – 8 hours. It appears that sertraline's peak plasma levels are lower in young males compared to young females.

The side effects of sertraline are dose related and tend to emerge at peak sertraline plasma levels after 6 – 8 hours. Further, the ingestion of sertraline with food results in the peak plasma level occurring within 5 hours rather than 8 hours when it is ingested on an empty stomach.

Steady state: The daily use of sertraline will result in steady plasma levels within 7 days.

Protein binding: 98%. In the serum, sertraline is highly bound to protein. It appears that more than 98% of the circulating sertraline is bound to albumin.

Half life (t 1/2): 26 – 32 hours for sertraline

70 Hours for *desmethylsertraline* (sertraline's principal metabolite).

Sertraline's relatively long half-life results in a lower incidence of discontinuation syndrome, as it takes at least seven days before sertraline is eliminated from the body.

Sertraline has a high lipid solubility and a small molecular size, which enables it to pass easily through the blood–brain barrier in high proportion. Studies on animals have shown that sertraline's concentration in the brain is 40 times higher than that in the blood.

Metabolism: Sertraline is primarily metabolized by the liver via the enzymes of the CYP450 system. The principal pathway of metabolism is N-demethylation.

N-desmethylsertraline, which is the active metabolite, has a plasma terminal half-life of 62 to 104 hours, but it appears to be less active than its parent drug.

N-desmethylsertraline has a 50 times weaker effect on SERT than that of the parent drug; practically, this metabolites has no clinical effects.

Both sertraline and N-desmethylsertraline subsequently undergo deamination, reduction, hydroxylation and glucuronide conjugation. The principal CYP 450 isoenzymes which are responsible for sertraline metabolism are:

- 2C9 (25%)
- 3A4 (15%)
- 2C19 (15%)
- 2D6 (5%)

Patients with liver disease can experience a significant decrease in sertraline metabolism, which can cause a *threefold increase* in sertraline's half-life.

Studies have shown that there are more than 80 genetic variants of the CYP 2D6 iso-enzymes. However, only 4 variants have been identified as responsible for poor metabolism of sertraline. Patients who have the poor metabolizing variant of the 2D6 enzyme may experience higher sertraline blood levels, similar to those with liver disease. Poor metabolizers and patients with a compromised liver require lower doses of sertraline to avoid excessive accumulation of the drug in the blood.

P-gp System

Sertraline is a **substrate** as well as a **strong inhibitor of the P-gp** functions in vivo and in vitro (1,2). The inhibitory effects of sertraline and N-desmethylsertraline on the P-gp system may interfere with the plasma levels of other co – administered drugs, which are P-gp substrates. It appears that the blood- brain barrier's P-gp system does not affect the entry of sertraline to the brain (8).

Elimination: Urine 0.2%, Faeces 50%. Sertraline is eliminated mainly by the **faeces.** Furthermore, studies on volunteers with mild, moderate and severe renal impairment revealed there the renal impairment had no effect on sertraline pharmacokinetics. The limited elimination of sertraline by the kidney enables patients with severe renal impairment to use sertraline safely without fear of drug accumulation.

How supplied

- Tablet: 25mg, 50mg, 100 mg
- Oral solution 20mg/ml

Dose range

- 50 mg – 200 mg for depression
- Doses of 200 mg a day may be required for OCD and bulimia

Sertraline clinical indications

- Major depressive disorder
- Panic disorder
- Obsessive compulsive disorder
- Premenstrual dysphoric syndrome
- Bulimia

OCD

Sertraline has been shown to be effective in the treatment of OCD independent of the patient's mood. In a double-blind randomized controlled study comparing sertraline to desipramine for concurrent OCD and depression, the patients on sertraline showed improvement in their OCD symptoms, and higher remission rates for MDD (6).

In addition, studies on children with OCD who were given sertraline also showed significant improvement over placebo. It appears that the OCD patients required the same dose of sertraline as patients with depression.

Major Depressive Disorder (MDD)

Several studies have established the superiority of sertraline over placebo in the treatment of major depression. Patients who were given sertraline at doses of 50mg – 200mg a day showed a significant improvement in their depressive symptoms at every dose level, and overall were significantly improved than with placebo.

There is no direct relationship between sertraline plasma concentration and the clinical response. Pooled data from 7 randomized controlled double blind studies comparing placebo and buproprion with the SSRIs fluoxetine, sertraline and paroxetine in outpatients with MDD showed no evidence for superior effectiveness of one SSRI over another while all drugs were superior to placebo (5). The results of a comparative study of the response and remission rates in MDD and OCD with the use of sertraline and desipramine are illustrated in Figure 17.1

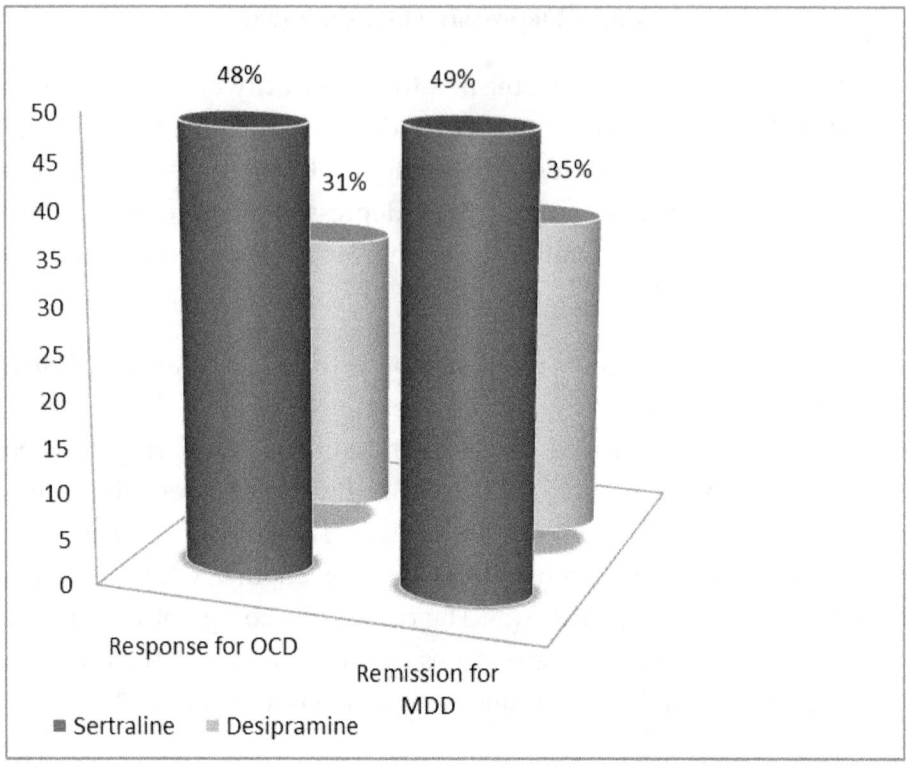

Figure 17.1 Response and Remission rates of sertraline and Desipramine in MDD and OCD. Adapted from Hoehn – Saric R, Ninan P, Black D. et al. Multicenter double blind comparison of sertraline and desipramine for concurrent OCD and MDD. Arch. Gen. Psychiatry 2000;57 (1): 76-82.

Furthermore, sertraline has been shown to have long-term efficacy. The recurrence of depression in patients receiving maintenance therapy with sertraline was only 13% versus 46% in those patients who received placebo (4).

Bulimia

In general, most agents capable of inhibiting SERT are efficacious in bulimia. Sertraline is one of the drugs of choice in the treatment of bulimia.

Panic disorder (PD)

It appears that all the SSRIs are effective in the treatment of PD. In a multi-centre outpatient study, patients with panic disorder without depression were randomized to either sertraline or placebo groups. The sertraline group showed a 77% reduction in the frequency of panic attacks compared to a 50% reduction for the placebo group(7).

Post Traumatic Stress Disorder (PTSD)

Sertraline has been shown to be effective for the treatment of PTSD both in the acute phase of the illness as well as in long-term use.

Premenstrual Dysphoric Disorder (PMDD)

Several studies with sertraline showed that sertraline has improved efficacy over placebo for the treatment of PMDD in doses of 50 - 100mg a day.

Social Anxiety Disorder

Sertraline is FDA approved drug for the treatment of social anxiety disorder.

How to treat with sertraline

- **For Depression & OCD:** Start with 50mg a day in a single morning dose. Wait at least two weeks to assess clinical improvement before increasing the dose in increments of 50 mg a week up to a maximum of 200mg a day.
- **For Panic disorder (PD), Social anxiety & Post-Traumatic Stress disorder (PTSD):** Start with sertraline 25mg a day, in order to avoid possible excitation and anxiety. Increase the dose in increments of 50mg after one week of treatment up to a maximum of 200mg a day. As a general rule, the higher the patient's anxiety is, the lower the starting dose of sertraline should be, and the slower the dose increase should be.
- **For premenstrual dysphoric disorder (PMDD):** Start with sertraline 50 mg a day, a week before the upcoming menses cycle. However, in severe cases, patients need to take the medication throughout the menstrual cycle.

When and how to take medication

Preferably, sertraline should be used during the morning in order to avoid insomnia, which may be develop whenever sertraline is taken at night.

How to stop sertraline

Due to its relatively long half-life, sertraline have lower incidence of withdrawal symptoms.

Reduce the dose of sertraline gradually with a 50% dose reduction every third day. In the event of the emergence of withdrawal symptoms, re-instate the previous dose of sertraline, and once the discontinuation symptoms disappear, reduce the sertraline dose in a smaller proportions and over a longer period.

How long it takes to get an antidepressant effect

In order to get an antidepressant effect, sertraline should be used daily for at least 2 – 4 weeks. Sertraline's efficacy may increase with dose increases. The majority of depressed patients experience the beneficial effects of sertraline at a dose of 100 mg a day. However, some patient require a higher dose, up to 200mg of sertraline a day, in order to have an adequate antidepressant effect.

Side effects of sertraline

The side effects of sertraline are most probably related to the increased serotonin levels in the brain and in other organs. Most side effects develop soon after the initiation of treatment with sertraline and often disappear with time. The most common side effects of sertraline are:

Nervous system

- Activation (infrequent)
- Insomnia
- Agitation
- Restlessness
- Jitteriness
- Anxiety
- Tremor
- Worsening motor symptoms of Parkinson's disease
- Increased sweating/ flushing
- Headache
- Dizziness
- Seizures (rare)
- Cognitive slowing
- Reduced attention
- Apathy

- Emotional blunting
- Rash

Gastro intestinal

The GI side effects are common with sertraline and can develop within 30 minutes of drug ingestion. It is possible that the GI side effects are more likely the result of the direct effect of sertraline on the intestinal mucosa than to its peak plasma levels.

- Decreased appetite
- Upper gastrointestinal symptoms
- Nausea
- Vomiting
- Dry mouth
- Diarrhea or constipation
- Possible weight loss

Sexual

Sertraline like all other SSRIs, may affect sexual desire, performance and satisfaction.

- Decreased sex drive
- Delayed ejaculation
- Impotence
- Inability to reach an orgasm

Suicide

The FDA requires all antidepressants to carry a black box warning stating that antidepressants may increase the risk of suicide in persons under the age of 25 years. This warning is based on data suggesting that suicidal ideations and behavior have a 2-fold increase in children and in adolescents, and a 1.5 –

fold increase in the 18 – 24 age group.

Sertraline side effects that require immediate attention

- Confusion
- Excitation
- Onset of seizure
- Yellow skin / eyes
- Severe allergic reaction
- Irregular heart beats
- Low blood pressure
- Bruising and bleeding (relatively rare)
- Induction of manic episode
- Activation of suicidal ideation and behaviour

Physical and psychological dependence

In animal studies, sertraline did not show abuse potential. Furthermore, in human clinical trials, there was no indication of drug seeking behaviour, euphoria and drug liking. However, sertraline can cause physical dependence, as evidenced by the presence of withdrawal symptoms upon abrupt discontinuation of the drug. This physical dependence on sertraline is similar to the other SNRIs and SSRIs. In general, clinicians should carefully monitor patients for signs of misuse or abuse.

Discontinuation reaction of sertraline

A sudden discontinuation of sertraline may be associated with a discontinuation reaction. The discontinuation symptoms are usually self-limiting. The most common symptoms of the sertraline discontinuation reaction are:

- Nausea
- insomnia
- dizziness

- light-headedness
- vertigo
- nightmares and vivid dreams
- sensation of electric shock in the body
- anxiety

Safety profile of sertraline

Use in pregnancy: Risk category C

Sertraline is not evidently teratogenic. In studies on rats that received 2 times the maximum recommended dose of sertraline, there was a dose-related increase of liver adenomas in male rats. Sertraline had no genotoxic effects in vivo and in vitro. Decreased in fertility was seen in rats that received 4 times the maximum recommended dose of sertraline.

The use of sertraline during the first trimester as well as throughout the pregnancy is not recommended.

Neonates exposed to sertraline late in the third trimester may develop complications soon after the delivery, which include respiratory distress, cyanosis, apnea, seizures, vomiting, hypoglycaemia, hypertonia, hyperreflexia, tremor, jitteriness, constant crying, temperature instability and feeding difficulties which may require subsequent prolonged hospitalization, respiratory support and tube feeding. In addition, newborns exposed to sertraline in late pregnancy have an increased risk for Persistent Pulmonary Hypertension of the Newborn (PPHN) which is associated with neonatal mortality.

Use during lactation

Sertraline is secreted into the breast milk. However, the amount of sertraline in the breast milk is unknown. Due to its unknown effects on the newborn's normal growth and development breast feeding should be avoided. However, in a woman who develops severe depression and suicidal ideation, during their pregnancy, the risk of using sertraline versus its benefits should be discussed with the patients.

Sertraline's drug interactions

Sertraline's drug interactions are due to its metabolism by the liver enzymes CYP 450 **2C9, 3A4, 2C19 and 2D6**.

Follows a list of sertraline's drug interactions with the possible clinical consequences.

- **Warfarin:** The concomitant use may displace warfarin from its protein carrier which may cause increased INR with possible risk of bleeding.
- **Phenytoin:** The concomitant use may result in increased phenytoin blood levels.
- **MAOI:** The concomitant use may result in CNS toxicity and serotonin syndrome. Patients must wait 21 days after MAOI was stopped before initiating treatment with sertraline. Patients that stop sertraline must wait 7 days before starting a MAOI.
- **Benzodiazepines:** The concomitant use may increase plasma levels of alprazolam, triazolam.
- **Buspirone:** The concomitant use may increase plasma levels of buspirone.
- **Lithium:** The concomitant use may increase tremor and nausea.
- **Pimozide & thioridazine:** The concomitant use may increase the plasma levels of both antipsychotic medications, which can cause cardiac arrhythmias.
- **Pindolol & Propranolol:** The concomitant use may increased their blood levels which results in higher rates of lethargy and bradycardia.

- **Analgesic:** The concomitant use may interfere with codeine's analgesic action.
- **LSD:** The concomitant use may cause grand mal seizures and worsening of flashbacks.
- **Immunosuppressants:** The concomitant use may **decrease cyclosporine clearance**.

Warnings for sertraline

- **Pregnancy:** Sertraline has an FDA risk category C. Try to avoid the use during pregnancy or breastfeeding. Assessment of the risks versus benefits must be discussed with the patient.
- **Myocardial infarction:** Sertraline is one of the few antidepressants that has been shown to be safe in the treatment of depression in patients with a history of myocardial infarction and angina.
- **Depressed pilots:** Sertraline was approved by the FAA for the treatment of depression in pilots.
- **Schizophrenic patients:** Sertraline has been shown to be effective in the treatment of depression in schizophrenic patients.
- **Children & adolescents:** Sertraline is effective in the treatment of depression in children and adolescents. Sertraline may increase the risk of suicidal thinking and behavior in children, adolescents and young adults aged 18-24. The use of antidepressants in this population must balance the risk of suicide with the clinical need. Careful monitoring of the patient's clinical worsening, and suicidality should also involve the family and all other caregivers.
- **Patients with increased prolactin levels:** Due to its minimal effect on prolactin, sertraline is effective in the treatment of depression in patients with high prolactin levels.

- **Hypomania & mania**: Activation of hypomania or mania occurred in 0.4% of sertraline treated patients.
- **Seizures**: No seizures were observed among 3000 patients treated with sertraline during sertraline FDA registration studies for MDD.
- **Discontinuation syndrome**: Discontinuation response may develop when sertraline is stopped abruptly. The most common discontinuation symptoms include dysphoric mood, agitation, anxiety, dizziness, irritability, paresthesias in the form of electric shock sensations, headaches, insomnia, emotional lability, lethargy and confusion. A gradual dose reduction is strongly recommended.
- **Hyponatremia**: Hyponatremia may develop subsequent to the use of sertraline, especially in volume depleted patients and in patients on diuretics. The symptoms of hyponatremia include headaches, reduced concentration, confusion, weakness and unsteadiness, which may lead to falls. Severe cases of hyponatremia may result in seizures, hallucinations respiratory arrest, coma and death.
- **Angle-closure glaucoma**: Sertraline may have an effect on pupil size, resulting in mydriasis. Patients with narrow-angle-glaucoma may experience increased intraocular pressure when treated with sertraline.
- **Abnormal bleeding**: Abnormal bleeding was observed in patients using sertraline. Concomitant use of warfarin, NSAIDs and aspirin may add to this risk.
- **Uricosuric effect:** A mean decrease of 7% in serum uric acid was observed in patients on sertraline.
- **Asymptomatic liver enzyme increase**: Asymptomatic increases in liver enzyme was reported in 0.8% of patients using sertraline within the first 9 weeks of treatment. Liver enzymes increase in patients on sertraline is clinically insignificant.

- **Elderly**: Sertraline needs a lower dose in the elderly.
- **Liver impairment**: Sertraline need a lower dose in patients with liver impairment.
- **MAOI:** Sertraline requires a 2-week washout period before starting with a MAOI. After stopping a MAOI, wait 21 days before starting sertraline.

Sertraline overdose

Sertraline *is rarely lethal in mono therapy overdose*. However, the concomitant use of sertraline with alcohol and /or with other central nervous depressants such as painkillers, barbiturates and benzo-diazepines, may result in death caused by respiratory depression.

General symptom progression of sertraline overdose

Initially, the patient might feel extremely tired and lethargic. The pulse will slow down, and the breathing frequency will also decrease. As the level of intoxication increases, the level of consciousness will decrease, and the patient will become unresponsive to external stimulations. The reflexes will disappear, and the breathing will get shallow. The patient's pulse and blood pressure will drop until cardiovascular system collapse.

Symptoms of sertraline over-dose are

- vomiting
- over-sedation
- somnolence
- dilated pupils
- abnormal heart rhythm
- tachycardia
- nausea
- tremor
- agitation

- coma
- seizures
- delirium
- hypertension / hypotension
- QTc prolongation
- syncope

Overdose management

In general, there is no antidote for sertraline overdose. Management is mainly supportive, aimed at maintaining respiration, pulse and blood pressure. In the event of a recent overdose with sertraline, a stomach washout with activated charcoal might help in the elimination of the un-absorbed drug and is done with a large bore oro-gastric tube with appropriate airway protection. The aim of the stomach lavage is to get rid of the drug leftovers.

In some ER departments, ipecac is also used in order to induce vomiting of the ingested toxin, however **induction of emesis is not recommended in semi-comatose and comatose patients**. Due to the large volume of distribution of sertraline, forced diuresis, dialysis hemo-perfusion and exchange transfusion are unlikely to be effective.

Keeping open the patient's airway is compulsory, especially in semi - comatose individuals. The patient should be placed on his side in order to prevent aspiration of the vomitus back to the lungs. Suffocation due to vomit is the leading cause of death in sertraline overdose.

Blood pressure and heart rate monitoring is very important. Fluid intake should be monitored with intra-venous infusion of saline and urinary output should also be carefully monitored.

In most cases, sertraline overdose, requires hospitalization of the patient for at least 24 hours for intense observation.

Sertraline references

1 Weiss J, Dormann SM, Martin- Facklam et al. Inhibition of P-gp by newer antidepressants. J. Pharmacol Exp Ther. Apr 2003; 305(1):197-204.

2 Akamine, Yumiko,Yasui-Furukori et al. Psychotropic drug – drug interactions involving P-gp. Nov 2012 Vol 26 issue 11- 959 – 973.

3 Hiemke C, Haarter S, et al. Pharmacokinetics of SSRI. Pharmacol Ther 2000;85:11 – 28.

4. Doogan DP, Caillard V et al. Sertraline in the prevention of depression. Br. J. Psychiatry 1992;160: 217-222.

5 Thase ME, Haight BR, Richard N. et al. Remission rates following antidepressant therapy with buproprion or SSRIs: A metaanalysis of original data from 7 randomized controlled trials. J. of Cl. Psy.2005; 66 (8): 974-981.

6 Hoehn – Saric R, Ninan P, Black D. et al. Multicenter double blind comparison of sertraline and desipramine for concurrent OCD and MDD. Arch. Gen. Psychiatry 2000;57 (1): 76-82.

7 Pohl R, Wolkow R, Clar C et al. Sertraline in the treatment of panic disorder: a double blind multicentre trial. Am J Psychiatry 1998;155: 1189-1195.

8 Jun-Sheng W, Hao-Jie Z. Bryan BG et al. Sertraline and its metabolite desmethylsertraline, but not Buproprion or its three major metabolites, have high affinity for P-gp. Biol Pharm Bull Feb 2008; 31(2): 231 – 234.

18
Tranylcypromine

Brand name: Parnate

Tranylcypromine's mode of action

Irreversible inhibition of MAO-A and MAO-B isoenzymes.

Tranylcypromine is a non-selective, irreversible inhibitor of both MAO- A & B isoenzymes. The inhibited enzymes become permanently inactive, and it takes 5-7 days until the neuron is capable of regenerating new enzymes. The inhibition of the MAO-A & B isoenzymes leads to the release of dopamine (DA), serotonin (5-HT) and norepinephrine (NE) into the synaptic region. The ability of tranylcypromine to release these neurotransmitters is approximately $1/10^{th}$ the potency of amphetamine. In addition, tranylcypromine can also increase the levels of tyramine, octopamine and tryptamine.

The selective effects of tranylcypromine on the anticholinergic, histaminergic and α adrenergic receptors are summarized as follows:

- ✓ **Anticholinergic Ach muscarinic affinity: Moderate.** Tranylcypromine has a moderate incidence of side effects which include dry mouth, constipation, blurred vision and drowsiness.

- ✓ **Histaminergic H1 affinity: Moderate.** Tranylcypromine has a moderate incidence of side effects which include sedation and weight gain.

✓ **α-1 adrenergic affinity: High.** Tranylcypromine has a high incidence of side effects which include hypotension, dizziness, drowsiness and other cardiovascular effects.

The MAO enzymes

There are two MAO isoenzyme in the body, namely MAO-A and MAO-B. Both isoenzymes are unequally distributed in the noradrenergic nerve cell terminals and are connected to the mitochondrial surface membrane.

In the body, the principal responsibility of the MAO enzymes is to regulate the quantities of the intracellular monoamines by means of deamination of the freely circulating plasma serotonin, norepinephrine and dopamine. The MAO isoenzymes are present in many tissues outside the central nervous system such as the intestinal epithelium and the liver.

MAO-A is the major isoenzyme present outside the brain, with the exception of the blood platelets which exclusively contain MAO-B. The distribution of the MAO enzymes in the body tissues is as follows:

- **MAO-A**: brain, gut, liver, skin,
- **MAO-B**: brain, platelets, lymphocytes

Both MAO isoenzymes are extensively distributed in the brain nerve cells. While MAO-A is predominantly distributed in the norepinephrine and the dopamine nerve cells, MAO-B is almost exclusively present in the serotonergic nerve cells. It appears that there is a clear-cut job description for the MAO enzymes, as each enzyme is responsible for metabolizing different intracellular monoamines.

➢ **MAO-A:** Is responsible for metabolizing the intracellular norepinephrine, serotonin, dopamine and tryptamine.

> **MAO-B** is responsible for metabolizing the intracellular dopamine, tryptamine, phenylethylamine, phenylethanolamine and tyramine.

The free intracellular biogenic monoamines are protected from the MAO enzyme action by their storage in a specific intracellular vesicle, distributed in the endoplasm of the presynaptic nerve terminals.

Each vesicle contains only one particular biogenic amine, such as dopamine, norepinephrine or serotonin. The free intracellular monoamines are actively transported from the cytoplasm into the vesicle by a special transporter called the VMAT. The body contains two VMAT isoforms, VMAT1 and VMAT2.

VMAT1 is located exclusively in the adrenal tissue, while VMAT2 is mostly distributed in the brain and in the enteric tissues.

It appears that the VMAT2 activity depends on the pH gradient between the cytoplasm and the intra-vesicular space. While the cytoplasm has a relative high pH, the intra-vesicle region has a lower pH, thus creating a pH gradient which serves as a driving force for the monoamine to be transported from the less acidic-cytoplasm into the vesicle.

VMAT-2 activity is inhibited by reserpine. Freed endoplasmatic monoamines are destroyed by the MAO enzymes, resulting in a lower level of monoamines to be released from the nerve terminals.

Chronic use of reserpine can lead to the depletion of the monoamine stores. Furthermore, there are other possible VMAT2 inhibitors such as tacrine, verapamil, estrogen and progesterone, which may cause monoamine depletion similar to that of reserpine and may contribute to the development of depression.

Tranylcypromine pharmacokinetics

Tranylcypromine has **non-linear pharmacokinetics** which implies that any dose-change leads to a dis-proportional change in the drug plasma levels. Regular tranylcypromine intake may result in higher than expected tranylcypromine plasma levels.

Peak plasma levels (Tmax): 1 – 2 hours.

Steady state: 5 -7 days of daily use. Steady plasma levels will result in a reduced risk of side effects. Substantial increases in 5-HT, DA and NE can be seen even though the parent compound has a very short half-life and is quickly eliminated from the body. This is due to the irreversible inhibition of the MAO-A & B enzymes and the need for at least 21 days to produce new MAO enzymes.

Absorption: Tranylcypromine is rapidly and well-absorbed by the gastrointestinal system. The rapid absorption of tranylcypromine is often correlated with abrupt increases in blood pressure and an abrupt rise in pulse rate.

Protein bound: Tranylcypromine is highly protein bound.

Bioavailability: 50%

Half-life (t ½): 2.5 hours A single dose of tranylcypromine will be quickly absorbed and will reach its peak plasma level within 1 -2 hours. However, the metabolism of tranylcypromine by the liver P-450 isoenzymes, and its steady elimination through the kidneys, results in a 50% reduction of the drug plasma levels after 2.5 hours.

Thus although tranylcypromine rapidly enters the blood, it is also quickly eliminated from it.

Metabolism: Tranylcypromine is primarily metabolised by the liver via the enzymes CYP450: **2A6, 2C19 and 2D6.**

The P-gp System

Tranylcypromine's effects on the **P-gp system are unknown.** However, it may have the potential to increase the bioavailability of co-administered P-gp substrates.

Elimination: Urine. Tranylcypromine is eliminated from the body mainly by the **urine** while only a small amount is eliminated by the faeces.

How supplied

- Tranylcypromine tablets: 10mg

Dose range

- Tranylcypromine 10mg – 60mg a day for the treatment of major depression

Tranylcypromine clinical indications

- Major depression (FDA approved)
- Treatment resistant depression
- Panic disorder

Major Depressive Disorder (MDD)

The efficacy of tranylcypromine for the treatment of depression is well established. Early studies suggested that tranylcypromine is especially effective for the treatment of atypical depression, characterized by the presence of depressed mood, anxiety, increased sleep and increased appetite. However, over the years tranylcypromine has been shown to be highly effective also in the treatment of major depression and in chronic resistant depressive patients. There is still some concern regarding the ability of tranylcypromine to induce mania in bipolar depressed patients, who therefore require close observation while on tranylcypromine in order to detect hypomania or mania.

Panic Disorder (PD)

Studies on patients with panic disorder have shown that tranylcypromine is effective in 60% of cases. The doses of tranylcypromine used in those trials were equal to those doses which were given to patients treated for major disorder.

When and how to take medication

Preferably take tranylcypromine in three divided doses of 10mg each in order to minimize the potential development of hypotension and tachycardia. As a general rule, always start with a low dose of 30mg a day and increase in a small proportions over a long period of time.

How to treat

For Major Depression (MDD): start treatment with tranylcypromine 30mg, a day preferably in divided doses. Slowly increase with increments of 10mg a day every seven days up to a maximum of 60mg/day which must be taken also in three divided doses.

How to stop tranylcypromine

Sudden termination of tranylcypromine use may be associated with the emergence of discontinuation symptoms. It is highly recommended to reduce the use of tranylcypromine slowly in order to minimize the emergence of withdrawal symptoms, which may develop within 1 - 4 days. The most recommended option is to reduce the dose of tranylcypromine by 50% every third day. However, in the event of the patient experiencing withdrawal symptoms, re-instate the previous dose of tranylcypromine, and once the discontinuation symptoms disappear, start tapering down the tranylcypromine dose in smaller proportions and over longer period of time.

How long it takes to get an antidepressant effect

The antidepressant effects of tranylcypromine require at least 7 – 28 days before a substantial mood improvement emerges.

Side effects of tranylcypromine

Most of the tranylcypromine side effects are probably related to its ability to increase serotonin, dopamine and norepinephrine levels in the brain.

The side effects are usually dose related and often develop soon after the initiation of treatment. They often correspond to the tranylcypromine peak plasma levels. In general, most side effects of tranylcypromine subside with time.

The most common side effects of tranylcypromine are:

Nervous system

- Drowsiness
- Lethargy, fatigue, weakness
- Dizziness
- Sedation
- insomnia
- Headache and worsening of migraine
- Disorientation
- Confusion
- Restlessness and agitation (rare)
- *Seizures* rare

- **Hypotension**
- Syncope
- tachycardia

Anticholinergic effects

- *Decreased appetite*
- *Dry mouth*
- Blurred vision
- Constipation
- Sweating
- Urinary retention

Gastro intestinal side effects: low incidence

- Nausea
- Vomiting

Sexual

- Decreased libido
- Impotence
- Retrograde ejaculation
- Delayed ejaculation

Tranylcypromine side effects that need immediate attention

- Confusion
- Excitation
- Onset of seizure
- Yellow skin / eyes
- Severe allergic reaction
- Irregular heart beat

- Hypotension
- Induction of manic or hypomanic episode
- Activation of suicidal ideation and suicidal behaviour especially in children and adolescents under the age of 25 years.

Suicide

The FDA requires all antidepressants to carry a black box warning stating that antidepressant may increase the risk for suicide in persons under the age of 25 years.

This warning is based on data suggesting that suicidal ideations and behavior has a 2-fold increase in children and in adolescents, and a 1.5 – fold increase in the 18 – 24 age group.

Physical & psychological dependence

There have been reports of drug dependency in patients using tranylcypromine in doses significantly in excess of the therapeutic range. Thus, patients with a history of drug abuse should be closely monitored for signs of tranylcypromine misuse or abuse, which include drug seeking behavior, development of tolerance and unsolicited dose increases as well as severe withdrawal symptoms that include restlessness, anxiety, headache, weakness, diarrhea, hallucinations and confusion.

Tranylcypromine discontinuation reaction

The sudden discontinuation of tranylcypromine may be associated with a discontinuation reaction. The discontinuation symptoms can develop within 1-3 days after the patient suddenly stops the use of tranylcypromine and can last up to three weeks. The discontinuation symptoms are usually self-limiting and eventually disappear.

The most common symptoms of tranylcypromine discontinuation reaction are

- Irritability
- Agitation
- Dizziness
- Anxiety
- Confusion
- Headache
- Lethargy
- Insomnia
- Seizures
- Dysphoric mood
- Fever
- Fatigue
- Sweating
- Myalgia (muscle pain)
- Hallucinations
- Vivid nightmares

A slow down titration of tranylcypromine can reduce the risk of having the discontinuation reaction.

Safety profile of tranylcypromine

Use in pregnancy: Risk category C

Tranylcypromine is not evidently teratogenic.

However, the use of tranylcypromine in the last trimester of pregnancy may be associated with higher incidence of respiratory distress and pulmonary hypertension, cyanosis, apnea, seizures, temperature instability vomiting, hypoglycemia, hypotonia, hyperreflexia, tremor, irritability, constant crying and jitteriness, with subsequent prolonged hospitalization, tube feeding and respiratory support.

There is an increased risk of the newborn to develop Persistent Pulmonary Hypertension of the Newborn (PPHN) and it is associated with substantial neonatal morbidity and mortality. Thus, the use of tranylcypromine during the first trimester as well as throughout the pregnancy is not recommended.

Use during lactation

Tranylcypromine is secreted in the breast milk. Due to its unknown effects on the newborn's normal growth and development, breast feeding should be avoided.

Carcinogenesis

There is no available information regarding carcinogenesis with the use of tranylcypromine.

Avoid using tranylcypromine in the following cases.

- **Myocardial infarction & cardiac impairment**: Patients who are recovering from myocardial infarction should avoid using tranylcypromine due its propensity to cause hypotension and tachycardia.
- **History of seizure**
- **Liver impairment**
- **Pheochromocytoma**
- **Presence of severe headache**
- **Anorexia & low body weight**
- **Proven allergy to tranylcypromine**
- **Co-administration with prohibited medications** (see drug interactions)
- **Co-administration with food containing high tyramine levels.** (See comprehensive list of food and beverages)
- **In patients who have a history of drug abuse- especially stimulants**

Tranylcypromine's drug interactions

Tranylcypromine's drug interactions usually occur with other drugs which are also substrates of the liver CYP 450 enzymes: **2A6, 2C19, 2D6**. The co-administration of other CYP 450 substrates may result in increased blood levels of tranylcypromine or of the competitive drug.

Follows a list of tranylcypromine's drug interactions with the consequent clinical reactions.

- **Tramadol:** The concomitant use may increase the risk of developing seizures.
- **Over the counter medications:** The concomitant use may cause **hypertensive crisis** when used in conjunction with: decongestants, antihistamine's, cough mixtures, narcotic, painkillers containing codeine, stimulants, appetite suppressants (fenfluramine and dexfenfluramine), and yeast dietary supplements.
- **All antidepressants:** The concomitant use may cause Serotonin syndrome. Wait 21 days after tranylcypromine was stopped before initiating treatment with another antidepressant. Wait at least 5-7 days before you starting tranylcypromine.
- **ACE – inhibitors, α 1 blockers, β blockers:** The concomitant use may enhance hypotension.
- **Buspiron:** The concomitant use may increase blood pressure.
- **Ginseng:** The concomitant use may cause headache.
- **L- tryptophan:** The concomitant use may cause **serotonin syndrome**.
- **Amphetamine, ephedrine, methylphenidate, pseudoephedrine, domapine, tyramine, adrenaline and salbutamol:** The concomitant use may cause **serotonin syndrome**.

- **Tryptans (sumatriptan, rizatriptan, zolmitriptan:** The concomitant use may cause **serotonin syndrome**.
- **Ecstasy:** The concomitant use may cause **serotonin syndrome**.

Tranylcypromine hypertensive crisis

Hypertensive crisis is a serious and dangerous medical condition which can develop when patients treated with tranylcypromine will consume a large amount of food that contains high levels of tyramine.

Tyramine is a natural monoamine compound which can be found in food and in plants. Tyramine can also be produced in food and beverages as a result of fermentation and spoilage.

Once ingested, tyramine gets absorbed through the gastro intestinal tract into the blood and distributes all over the body with the exception of the brain as the tyramine molecule is unable to cross the blood-brain barrier. In the human body, tyramine induces the release of dopamine (DA) and norepinephrine (NE) which can cause vasoconstriction and high blood pressure.

In regular circumstances, the MAO-A enzyme, located inside the cells, controls the amount of norepinephrine and dopamine, by the breaking down the excess neurotransmitters.

This normally results in controlled blood pressure.

However, in a patient on tranylcypromine who ingests a large amount of tyramine, the irreversible inhibition of MAO-A enzymes, by MAOI results in a disproportionate increase in norepinephrine and dopamine. This then stimulates the α1 adrenergic receptors in the blood vessel endothelium, causing vasoconstriction and elevated blood pressure.

Food containing tyramine is absorbed through the intestinal wall and gets destroyed immediately by the gastroenteric MAO-A enzymes which act like gate keepers. However, there is always a small amount of tyramine which may escape and leak into the blood stream.

Nevertheless, the second line of defense which protects the body from too much tyramine in the blood is the liver, which is also capable of destroying the free tyramine with its own MAO-A enzymes.

In normal situations, the MAO-A enzyme can handle food containing up to **400mg** of ingested tyramine before any change in blood pressure develops. A high tyramine content meal contains approximately **40mg** of tyramine, which is easily destroyed by the MAO-A enzymes.

However, in the patient on tranylcypromine, the majority of its MAO-A enzyme is inhibited, resulting in limited ability to handle the excess in tyramine, and increasing the patient's vulnerability to develop elevated blood pressures.

Thus, patients on tranylcypromine that consume a meal containing as little as 10mg of tyramine may develop a significant and sudden increase in their blood pressure. Hypertensive crisis is a surge in blood pressure, which may exceed 180/120mm Hg. Hypertensive crisis is a medical emergency that may cause intracranial bleeding and death.

Hypertensive crisis is divided into two categories: Hypertensive urgency and hypertensive emergency.

> - **Hypertensive urgency**: is an acute elevation in blood pressure without end-organ damage.

> **Hypertensive emergency**: is an acute elevation in blood pressure which is accompanied by end-organ damage. Hypertensive emergency can be associated with life-threatening complications such as brain hemorage and organs failure.

Causes of hypertensive emergency include

- Poor compliance of blood pressure medications.
- Myocardiac infarction
- Heart failure
- Kidney failure
- Stroke
- Eclampsia
- Food containing high levels of tyramine.

Despite the possible risk of developing hypertensive crisis from foods containing tyramine, tranylcypromine users can still enjoy some foods containing tyramine. For example, one needs to eat more than 20 pieces of pizza or drink the same number of wine or beer glasses before the patient is at risk of developing hypertensive crisis (3).

The physiological effects of incremental tyramine intake in patients using tranylcypromine are as follows:

> **Tyramine 8mg**: Elevated blood pressure, increased heart rate.
> **Tyramine 10mg**: Headache, nausea, vomiting.
> **Tyramine 25mg**: Hypertensive crisis.

The clinical symptoms of hypertensive crisis characterized by the sudden onset of occipital headache, which may radiate frontally, palpitation, neck stiffness, neck pain, nausea, vomiting, sweating, and photophobia. In addition, the patient may experience chest pain, tachycardia and pupil dilation. The cardiac findings of hypertensive crisis include prominent apical pulsation and cardiac enlargement. The funduscopic findings of hypertensive crisis may include papilledema and hemorrhages. Most patients present with blood pressure that exceeds 180/120 mm Hg, which may lead to intracranial bleeding with a fatal outcome.

Hypertensive crisis requires immediate discontinuation of tranylcypromine, as well as therapy to lower blood pressure. These should be given immediately and slowly titrated in order to avoid an excessive drop in blood pressure. Excessive blood pressure lowering should be avoided due to the risk of getting cerebral ischemia if blood pressure falls too quickly.

Oral antihypertensive medication includes:

- ACE inhibitors,
- Beta-blockers
- Calcium channel blocker.

Patient may be observed for several hours and once their blood pressure returns to normal levels they can be followed up as outpatient. Patients with hypertensive emergency should be admitted to an intensive care for close monitoring of hemodynamics, urine output and of other ends-organ damages.

Symptoms of hypertensive crisis are

- Occipital headache,
- Neck stiffness
- Nausea
- Vomiting
- Dilated pupils and photophobia
- Bleeding nose
- Chest pain

- Tachycardia
- Shortness of breath
- Seizures
- Unresponsiveness

Hypertensive crisis is a medical emergency which requires immediate medical intervention with the aim to reduce the elevated blood pressure which may have catastrophic consequences.

Food restrictions when using tranylcypromine

Due to the danger of the serious interactions of tranylcypromine with food containing tyramine, the amount of ingested tyramine must be strictly controlled. Follows a list of food and their tyramine content.

Food containing high levels of tyramine which should be avoided

- All matured aged cheeses: cheddar, blue, Roquefort, camembert
- Marmite
- Broad beans
- Pickled herring & other dried fish
- Soups in packets
- Sauerkraut
- Aged smoked meat
- Beer
- Wine
- Liver
- Hard salami
- Dried sausage
- Pepperoni
- Yogurt

- Tofu

Food containings low tyramine levels which can be ingested in moderation

- Cottage cheese
- Sour cream
- Salad dressing

As a general rule, fresh food has a low tyramine content, while spoiled and processed food, canned food, gravy sauces and fermented food contain higher levels of tyramine.

Warnings for tranylcypromine

- **Pregnancy: Risk category C.** Try to avoid use during pregnancy or breastfeeding. Assessment of the risks versus benefits must be discussed with the patient.
- **Tranylcypromine may cause an increase in suicidal risk in young adults.** Tranylcypromine, as all antidepressants used for MDD may increase the risk of suicidal thinking and behavior in children, adolescents and young adults aged 18-24. The use of antidepressants in this population must balance the risk of suicide with the clinical need. Careful monitoring of the patient's clinical worsening, and suicidality should also involve the family and all other caregivers.
- **Activation of hypomania or mania** may occur in tranylcypromine treated bipolar patients. As tranylcypromine may trigger mania in predisposed patients, it should be used cautiously in patients with a history of bipolar mood disorder
- **Serotonin syndrome** may develop with tranylcypromine use. Symptoms of serotonin syndrome may include agitation, dizziness, hallucinations, delirium, seizures and coma along with autonomic instability including

tachycardia, fluctuating blood pressure, flushing, hyperthermia, tremor, muscular rigidity, myoclonus, hyperreflexia, incoordination. The concomitant use of tranylcypromine with antidepressants and triptans may precipitate serotonin syndrome which may be fatal.
- **Over-the-counter medications:** Tranylcypromine use combined with many psychotropic and other over the counter medications may cause serotonin syndrome.
- **Syncope:** Tranylcypromine use was associated with syncope and hypotension. Postural hypotension may be relieved by having the patient lie down with their legs elevated until blood pressure returns to normal. The concomitant use of tranylcypromine with anti-hypertensive drugs may exacerbate hypotension.
- **Heart disease:** Tranylcypromine may have the capacity to suppress angina pain that would otherwise serve as a warning sign for myocardial ischemia. Further, Tranylcypromine is not recommended for use during the initial phase of myocardial infarction as it is associated with QT prolongation and isolated PVCs, tachycardia, syncope and torsades de pointes. Finally, tranylcypromine needs to be used with caution in patients with cardiac impairment and should be avoided in patients who recently had a myocardial infarct.
- **Kidney dysfunction.** Tranylcypromine requires a lower dose adjustment in patients with kidney impairment due to its elimination in the urine.
- **Liver dysfunction.** Tranylcypromine requires a lower dose adjustment in patients with liver dysfunction due to its extensive metabolism by the liver CYP 450 enzymatic system.
- **Elderly:** Tranylcypromine needs a lower dose adjustment in the elderly.

> **Seizure:** Tranylcypromine may lower the seizure threshold, thus suitable precautions should be taken in patients with history of seizures..
> **Alcohol abuse:** Tranylcypromine is not recommended in patients abusing alcohol. In addition, tranylcypromine should be used with caution in patient using disulfiram (antabuse). A study on rats which were given high doses of tranylcypromine plus Antabuse experienced severe toxicity including convulsions and death.

Tranylcypromine overdose

Tranylcypromine **can be lethal in mono therapy overdose**, which may result in a high incidence of fatalities. Moreover, the concomitant use of tranylcypromine with alcohol and/ or with other central nervous depressants such as painkillers or benzodiazepines may result in death cause by the additive effects of the combined medications on the patient's respiratory system causing respiratory depression and cardio-respiratory arrest, metabolic acidosis and hypoxia.

A patient overdosed on tranylcypromine may be symptom free for up to six hours after tranylcypromine ingestion. Only later may they become restless and comatose. Therefore, close medical monitoring is required for at least 48 hours following tranylcyprominr overdose.

General symptoms of tranylcypromine overdose

Initially, the patient might feel extremely tired and lethargic. The pulse will slow down, and the breathing frequency will also decrease. As the level of intoxication increases, the level of consciousness will decrease, and the patient will become unresponsive to external stimulations. The reflexes will disappear, and the breathing will get shallow. The patient's pulse and blood pressure will drop until cardiovascular system collapse.

The most common symptoms of tranylcypromine overdose are

- over sedation
- respiratory arrest
- seizure
- abnormal heart rhythm – mainly tachycardia
- hypotension
- vomiting
- ataxia
- headache
- restlessness
- confusion
- delirium
- loss of consciousness

What to do in the case of tranylcypromine overdose

In general, there is no antidote for tranylcypromine overdose. Management is mainly supportive, aimed at maintaining respiration, pulse and blood pressure. In the event of a recent overdose with tranylcypromine, a stomach washout with activated charcoal might help in the elimination of the unabsorbed drug and is done with a large bore oro-gastric tube with appropriate airway protection. The aim of the stomach lavage is to get rid of the drug leftovers.

In some ER departments, ipecac is also used in order to induce vomiting of the ingested toxin, however **induction of emesis is not recommended in semi-comatose and comatose patients**. Due to the large volume of distribution of tranylcypromine, forced diuresis, dialysis hemo-perfusion and exchange transfusion are unlikely to be effective. Keeping open the patient's airway is compulsory, especially in semi - comatose individuals. The patient should be placed on his side in order to prevent aspiration of the vomitus back to the lungs. Suffocation due to vomit is the leading cause of death in tranylcypromine overdose. Blood pressure and heart rate monitoring is very important. Fluid intake should be monitored with intra -venous infusion of saline and urinary output should be also carefully monitored. In most cases, tranylcypromine overdose, requires hospitalization of the patient for at least 48 hours for intense observation.

Tranylcypromine references

1 Akamine, Yumiko,Yasui-Furukori et al. Psychotropic drug – drug interactions involving P-gp. Nov 2012 Vol 26 issue 11- 959 – 973.

2 Weiss j, Dormann SM, Martin- Facklam et al. Inhibition of P-gp by newer antidepressants. J. Pharmacol Exp Ther. Apr 2003;; 305(1):197-204.

3 SM Stahl. Stahl's Essential Psychopharmacology, Third edition. Cambridge University Press 2008.

19

Trazodone

Brand names:

Desyrel

Molipaxin

Oleptro

Mode of action: Trazodone

1. Trazodone is a weak antagonist of the Serotonin Reuptake Transporter (SERT): The inhibition by trazodone, of the SERT located on the presynaptic neurons, results in increased serotonin synaptic levels. Trazodone's ability to inhibit SERT is much weaker compared to other SSRIs.

2. Trazodone is a strong *agonist* of the post-synaptic 5-HT 1A receptors:

The activation of the 5-HT1A post-synaptic receptor *stimulates* the release of dopamine which has a favourable antidepressant effect as well as a positive effects on anxiety and cognition.

3. Trazodone a post-synaptic 5-HT2A receptor antagonist:

The inhibition of the post-synaptic 5-HT2A receptors has been implicated in trazodone's antidepressant effect by stimulating the release of cortical dopamine.

4. Trazodone is a post-synaptic 5-HT2C receptor antagonist:

The inhibition of the post-synaptic 5-HT2C receptors *regulates* the release of cortical dopamine and noradrenaline, both of which are involved in depression, emotions, concentration and weight.

The selective effects of trazodone on the anticholinergic, histaminergic and α adrenergic receptors are summarized as follows:

- ✓ **Anticholinergic Ach muscarinic affinity: High.** Trazodone has a high incidence of side effects of dry mouth, constipation, blurred vision and drowsiness.

- ✓ **Histaminergic H1 affinity: Moderate.** Trazodone has a moderate incidence of side effects of sedation and weight gain.

- ✓ **α 1 adrenergic affinity: Moderate.** Trazodone has a moderate incidence of side effects of hypotension, dizziness, drowsiness and other cardiovascular effects.

Pharmacokinetics of trazadone

Absorption: Trazodone has **linear pharmacokinetics** and it does not appears to induce its own metabolism. Thus, any dose change leads to a proportional change in the drug plasma levels. Trazodone is well absorbed by the gastrointestinal system. However, the absorption of trazodone is *slowed by the presence of food* in the stomach, which may result in a delayed increase in trazodone plasma levels.

Peak plasma levels (T_{max}): 1 hour for trazodone

43 hours for the metabolite m-CPP

Trazodone side effects tend to emerge at the peak of its plasma level. A single dose of trazodone may result in side effects within 1 hour of drug ingestion.

Steady state: 3 – 7 days. Daily use of trazodone will lead to steady plasma levels within 3 -7 days and is often associated with a significant reduction in side effects.

Although the parent compound has a very short half- life, the active metabolite m-CPP has a much longer half-life which somewhat reduces the risk of discontinuation syndrome. However, it is still prudent to taper down slowly trazodone when considering stopping trazodone.

Trazodone elimination half- life (t 1/2):

>9 hours for trazodone.

>4 -14 hoursfor m-CPP

Protein binding: 95%. Trazodone is highly protein bound to the plasma albumin.

Metabolism: Trazodone is primarily metabolised by the liver via the enzyme CYP450: **3A4.**

Trazodone has an active metabolite called **m-CPP** which can accumulate to higher levels in the brain than in the blood. More than 75% of trazodone metabolites are excreted within 3 days. However, patients with liver disease can experience a significant decrease in trazodone metabolism, which may cause trazodone to accumulate in the blood. Thus, trazodone should be avoided in patients with compromised livers as well as heavy alcohol abusers.

The P-gp System

Trazodone is a P-gp inhibitor (3), and may have the potential to increase the bioavailability of co-administered compounds that are substrates of P-gp. In addition, the concentration of trazodone in the intestine after chronic oral dosing may induce the expression of intestinal P-gp and consequently reduce the absorption of co-administered drugs (3).

Elimination: Urine 80%, Faeces 20%.

Dose range

- Trazodone 150 mg–400mg a day for depression
- Trazodone XR 150mg–375mg a day for depression

How supplied

- Trazodone immediate release tablets 50mg, 100mg. 150mg
- Trazodone XR 150mg, 300mg

How to treat

- **For Major Depressive Disorder** Start with trazodone 150mg in divided doses to be increased every 3 days to a maximum of 400mg in divided doses.

- For the treatment of depression with the extended release formula (trazodone XR), start with trazodone XR 150mg once a day to be increased every 3 days by 75 mg to a maximum dose of 375mg.

- **For insomnia** Start with trazodone 50 mg in the evening, to be increased up to 100mg at bedtime.

When and how to take medication

Preferably take trazodone twice a day for the immediate release formulation and once a day at bedtime for the XR formulation. In general use the principle "start low and go slow", as patients can experience over-sedation the following day at the beginning of the treatment.

Clinical indications

- Major depression
- insomnia
- anxiety

Major Depressive Disorder (MDD)

The efficacy of trazodone in the treatment of MDD showed comparable efficacy to that of other tricyclic antidepressants, and a better efficacy than placebo (4). Trazodone's response rates compared to amitryptiline and placebo are illustrated in figure 19.1

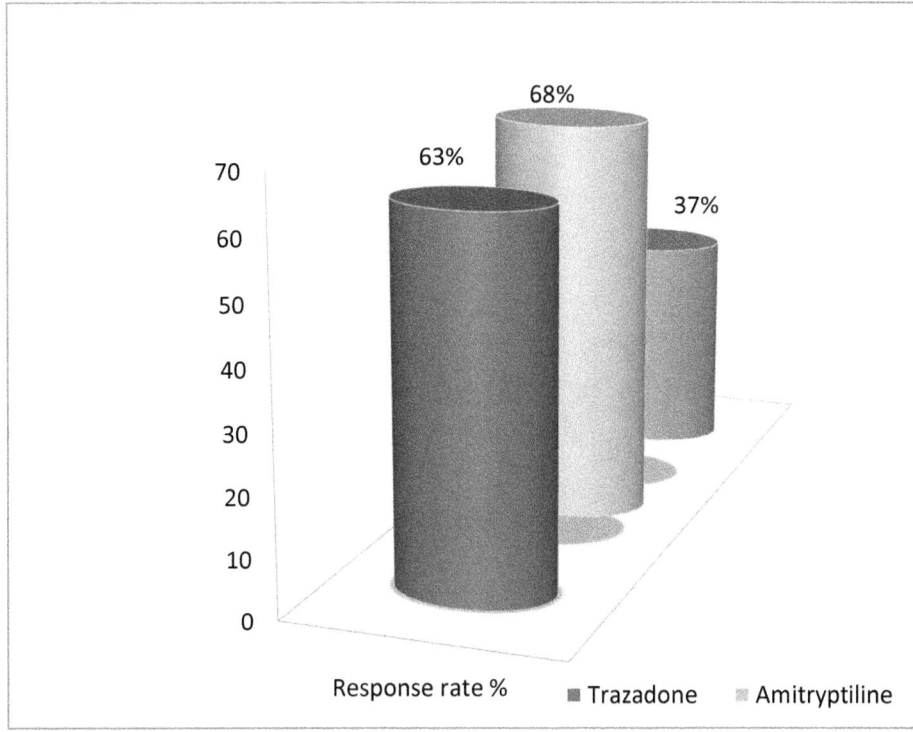

Figure 19.1: Trazodone response rate compared to amitryptiline and placebo. Adapted from Goldberg HL, Rickels K, Finnely R. Treatment of depression with a new antidepressant. J Clin Psychopharmacology. 1981; sup. 6 , 1:3s- 38s.

However, in a double blind placebo-controlled study of trazodone, venlafaxine and placebo, trazodone showed a lower efficacy rate of 60% compared to venlafaxine's efficacy rate of 72%.

Both were significantly more efficacious than placebo (efficacy rate 55%) (5) as illustrated in Figure 19.2.

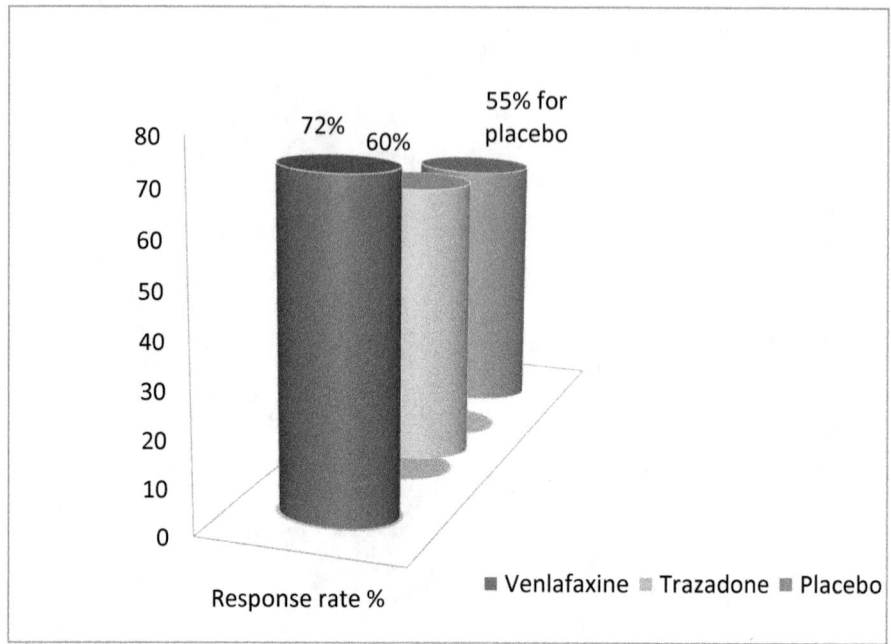

Figure 19.2: Trazodone's response rate compared with venlafaxine and placebo. Adapted from Cunningham LA, Borison RL, Carman JS et al. A comparison of venlafaxine, trazodone and placebo in MDD. J Clin Psychopharmacology 1994;14:99-106.

Studies in the depressed geriatric population showed that trazodone has significant efficacy. However, trazodone's side effects of severe sedation and low blood pressure may cause severe dizziness with an increased risk of falls, which may have catastrophic clinical implications (5). Therefore, trazodone's use among the elderly is less acceptable.

Anxiety

Trazodone has been reported to have significant antianxiety properties. The antianxiety effects of trazodone are comparable to that of diazepam.

Insomnia

Trazodone can be used in a low dose as an alternative to sleeping medications. A recent survey among clinicians reported that 78% of psychiatrists prefer to use trazodone for SSRI- induced insomnia (6).

Safety profile of trazodone

Use in pregnancy: Risk category C

Trazodone is not evidently teratogenic.

No teratogenic effects were seen in studies performed in rats at doses 50 times the maximum recommendedhuman dose (MRHD). However, the use of trazodone in the last trimester of pregnancy is associated with a higher incidence of respiratory distress and pulmonary hypertension, cyanosis, apnea, seizures, temperature instability vomiting, hypoglycemia, hypotonia, hyperreflexia, tremor, irritability, constant crying and jitteriness, which subsequently required prolonged hospitalization, tube feeding and respiratory support. There is an increased risk of the newborn developing Persistent Pulmonary Hypertenion (PPHN) which is associated with substantial neonatal morbidity and mortality. Thus, the use of trazodone during the first trimester as well as throughout the pregnancy is not recommended.

Carcinogenesis

There is no evidence of carcinogenesis with the use of trazodone in treated rats with daily doses up to 300mg/kg for 18 months.

Use during lactation

Trazodone is secreted in the breast milk. Due to its unknown effects on the newborn's normal growth and development breast feeding should be avoided.

Avoid using trazodone in the following cases:

- **Priapism:** In the event of male patients getting a painful erection which lasts longer than 4-6 hours, immediate urgent medical help is required. Priapism is often self-limited and reverses spontaneously. However, in 30% of cases, it requires surgical intervention which may cause permanently impaired erectile function or impotence.
- **Persistent genital arousal in female:** Persistent genital arousal may be associated with trazodone use in female patients and it is similar to male priapism.
- **Cardiac arrhythmia:** Patients with pre-existing cardiac disease and cardiac arrhythmias should be closely monitored.
- History of seizure
- Proven allergy to trazodone

How to stop trazodone

Although the incidence of withdrawal symptoms following trazodone cessation is relatively low, a slow tapering of trazodone is recommended. In the event of getting withdrawal symptoms, re-instate the previous dose, and once the symptoms disappear, start reducing the trazadone dose in smaller proportions and over longer period of time.

How long it takes to get an antidepressant effect

Like all antidepressants trazodone needs at least 7 – 28 days before a substantial mood improvement emerges.

Trazodone drug interactions

Follows a list of trazodone drug interactions.

- **Digoxin:** The concomitant use may cause higher digoxin blood levels.

- **Grapefruit juice interaction:** The concomitant use may decrease trazodone metabolism.
- **St John's Wort:** The concomitant use may cause serotonin syndrome.
- **Ginko biloba:** The concomitant use may cause **coma.**
- **Phenytoin:** The concomitant use may cause higher phenytoin blood levels.
- **Tramadol:** The concomitant use may cause seizures.
- **Fluoxetine:** The concomitant use may cause increase in trazodone blood levels.
- **Clonidine:** The concomitant use may interfere with clonidine's antihypertensive effects.
- **MAOI:** The concomitant use may cause CNS toxicity-serotonin syndrome. Wait 21 days after the MAOI was stopped before initiating treatment with trazodone. Wait 5-7 days after discontinuing trazodone before starting a MAOI.
- **Carbamazepine:** The concomitant use may decrease trazodone plasma levels.
- **Zolpidem:** The concomitant use may cause increased sedation.
- **Alprazolam:** The concomitant use may increase alprazolam blood concentrations by 200%.
- **Clozapine:** The concomitant use may lead to increased clozapine blood levels.
- **Sildenafil:** The concomitant use may enhance hypotension.
- **Simvastatin, pravastatin, atorvastatin:** The concomitant use may increase statin plasma levels with increased risk of harmful side effects including myositis and rhabdomyolysis.

Side effects of trazodone

Most side effects of trazodone are probably related to its ability to increase serotonin in the brain as well as its inhibitory effects on α1 adrenergic receptors and H1 receptors, which often results in hypotension (with α1) and over sedation (with H1). The side effects related to trazodone are usually dose-related and often develop soon after the initiation of treatment, and subside with time. The most common side effects of trazodone are:

Nervous system

- Drowsiness
- Lethargy
- Fatigue
- Weakness
- Dizziness
- Sedation
- Nausea
- Blurred vision
- Headache and worsening of migraine
- In coordination
- Tremor
- Disturbed concentration
- Disorientation
- Confusion
- Restlessness and agitation (rare)
- *Seizures* (more common in predisposed individuals, if occur, is often after sudden drug dose increase or after drug withdrawal).
- Stuttering
- Disturbance in gait
- Worsening of parkinsonism
- Rash (rare 1%)

- Hypotension
- Syncope
- bradycardia

Gastro intestinal

The gastro intestinal side effects of trazodone can develop within 30 minutes of drug ingestion and they are more likely the result of the trazodone's effects on serotonin uptake and its anticholinergic effects.

- *Decreased appetite*
- Weight gain
- Nausea
- Vomiting
- Dry mouth
- Glossitis
- Strange taste in mouth
- Constipation
- Gastritis

Sexual

- Increased libido
- Priapism
- Spontaneous orgasm with yawning
- Retrograde ejaculation
- Painful ejaculation
- Testicular swelling

Trazodone's side effects that need immediate attention

- Priapism
- Confusion
- Excitation

- Onset of seizure
- Yellow skin / eyes
- Severe allergic reaction
- Irregular heart beats
- Hypotension
- Induction of manic or hypomanic episode
- Activation of suicidal ideation and behaviour especially in children and adolescents

Trazodone's discontinuation reaction

The sudden discontinuation of trazodone may be associated with a discontinuation reaction which occurs in 20% – 80% of treated patients. The discontinuation symptoms are usually self limiting.

The most common symptoms of trazodone's discontinuation reaction are

- Irritability
- Agitation
- Dizziness
- Anxiety
- Confusion
- Headache
- Lethargy
- Insomnia
- Seizures
- Dysphoric mood
- Fever
- Fatigue
- Sweating
- Myalgia (muscle pain)
- Priapism

A slow down-titration of trazodone's often reduces the risk of having the discontinuation reaction.

Suicide

The FDA requires all antidepressants to carry a black box warning stating that antidepressants may increase the risk for suicide in persons under the age of 25 years. This warning is based on data suggesting that suicidal ideations and behavior has a 2-fold increase in children and in adolescents, and a 1.5- fold increase in the 18 – 24 age group.

Warnings for trazodone

- **Pregnancy: Risk category C.** Try to avoid use during pregnancy or breastfeeding. Assessment of the risks versus benefits must be discussed with the patient.
- **Trazodone may cause an increase in suicidal risk in young adults.** The use of antidepressants in this population must balance the risks of suicide with the clinical need. Careful monitoring of the patient's clinical worsening is necessary, and monitoring for suicidality should also involve the family and all other caregivers.
- **Activation of hypomania or mania** may occur in trazodone treated bipolar patients. As trazodone may trigger mania in predisposed patients, it should be used cautiously in patients with a history of bipolar mood disorder.
- **Serotonin syndrome** may develop with trazodone use. Serotonin syndrome symptoms may include agitation, dizziness, hallucinations, delirium, seizures and coma along with autonomic instability which includes tachycardia, fluctuating blood pressure, flushing, hyperthermia, tremor, muscular rigidity, myoclonus, hyperreflexia, and incoordination. The concomitant use of

trazodone with a MAOI may precipitate serotonin syndrome, which may be fatal.
- **MAOI:** After stopping trazodone a **7 day** washout period is needed before starting with a MAOI. After the MAOI was stopped, a **3 week** washout period is necessary before starting trazodone.
- **Priapism**: Painful erections lasting longer than 6 hours were reported in men taking trazodone. Priapism, if not treated promptly, may result in irreversible damage to the erectile tissue. Patients with anatomical deformation of the penis (such as cavernosal fibrosis, angulation or Peyronie's disease), as well as patients with sickle cell anemia, multiple myeloma or leukemia, should use trazodone with care as those conditions may predispose them to priapism. Patients who develop priapism lasting longer than 6 hour should seek emergency medical attention.
- **Hyponatremia:** Hyponatremia may develop subsequent to the use of trazodone, especially in volume depleted patients and in patients on diuretics. The symptoms of hyponatremia include headaches, reduced concentration, confusion, weakness and unsteadiness, which may lead to falls. Severe cases of hyponatremia may result in seizures, hallucinations respiratory arrest, coma and death.
- **Abnormal bleeding** was observed in patients using trazodone. Concomitant use of warfarin, NSAIDs aspirin may add to this risk.
- **Syncope:** Trazodone use was associated with syncope and hypotension. The concomitant use of trazodone with anti-hypertensive drugs may exacerbate hypotension.
- **Angle–closure glaucoma**: Trazodone may have an effect on pupil size resulting in mydriasis. Patients with narrow-angle glaucoma may experience increased intraocular pressure when treated with trazodone.

- ➤ **Cognitive & motor impairment**: Trazodone may cause somnolence and sedation, which may impair the mental and the physical ability required for the performance of hazardous tasks.
- ➤ **Discontinuation symptoms:** Trazodone discontinuation was associated with withdrawal symptoms of anxiety, agitation, and sleep disturbances. A gradual dose reduction is strongly recommended in order to avoid discontinuation symptoms.
- ➤ **Heart disease**: Trazodone is not recommended for use during the initial phase after having a myocardial infarction. Trazodone was associated with QT prolongation and isolated PVCs, tachycardia, syncope and torsade de pointes.
- ➤ **Liver impairment**: Trazodone should be taken in a lower dose in people with liver cirrhosis. Trazodone *must be avoided* in patients with liver insufficiency.
- ➤ **Alcohol abuse**: Trazodone is not recommended in patients abusing alcohol.
- ➤ **Kidney impairment**: Trazodone requires a dose adjustment (lower dose) in mild to moderate renal impairment.
- ➤ **Elderly:** Trazodone needs a dose adjustment (lower dose) in the elderly.

Physical & psychological dependence

Trazodone did not show any tendencies for drug seeking behaviour. However, patients with a history of drug abuse should be closely monitored for signs of trazodone misuse or abuse, which includes drug seeking behavior, development of tolerance and unmonitored dose increases.

Trazodone overdose

General symptoms of trazodone overdose

Initially, the patient might feel extremely tired and lethargic. The pulse will slow down, and the breathing frequency will decrease. As the level of intoxication increases, the level of consciousness will decrease, and the patient will become unresponsive to external stimulations. The reflexes will disappear, and the breathing will get shallow. The patient's pulse and blood pressure will drop until cardiovascular system collapse

Trazodone is relatively safe in mono therapy overdose with a rare incidence of fatalities. However, the concomitant use of trazodone with alcohol and with other central nervous depressants such as painkillers or benzo-diazepines may result in death caused by respiratory depression. The possible fatalities are often the result of cardio-respiratory arrest or the metabolic acidosis and hypoxia associated with status epilepticus.

Symptoms of trazodone over dose

- Over-sedation
- respiratory arrest
- seizure
- abnormal heart rhythm – mainly tachycardia
- hypotension
- priapism
- vomiting
- delirium
- loss of consciousness

What to do in the case of trazodone overdose

In general, there is no antidote for trazodone overdose. Management is mainly supportive, aimed at maintaining respiration, pulse and blood pressure. In the event of a recent overdose with trazodone a stomach washout with activated charcoal might help in the elimination of the un-absorbed drug and is done with a large bore oro-gastric tube with appropriate airway protection. The aim of the stomach lavage is to get rid of the drug leftovers.

In some ER departments, ipecac is also used in order to induce vomiting of the ingested toxin, however **induction of emesis is not recommended in semi-comatose and comatose patients**. Due to the large volume of distribution of trazoadone, forced diuresis, dialysis hemo-perfusion and exchange transfusion are unlikely to be effective. Keeping open the patient's airway is compulsory, especially in semi - comatose individuals. The patient should be placed on his side in order to prevent aspiration of the vomitus back to the lungs. Suffocation due to vomit is the leading cause of death in trazodone overdose. Blood pressure and heart rate monitoring is very important. Fluid intake should be monitored with intra -venous infusion of saline, and urinary output should be also carefully monitored. In most cases, trazodone overdose, requires hospitalization of the patient for at least 24 hours for intense observation.

Trazodone references

1 Akamine, Yumiko,Yasui-Furukori et al. Psychotropic drug – drug interactions involving P-gp. Nov 2012 Vol 26 issue 11- 959 – 973.

2 Weiss j, Dormann SM, Martin- Facklam et al. Inhibition of P-gp by newer antidepressants. J. Pharmacol Exp Ther. Apr 2003; 305(1):197-204.

3 Stormer EE,Von Moltke LL, Perkoff MD et al. P-gp interactions of nefazodone and trazodone in cell culture. J Clin Pharmacology 2001, 41 (7):708-714.

4 Goldberg HL,Rickels K, Finnely R. Treatment of depression with a new antidepressant. J Clin Psychopharmacology. 1981; sup. 6 , 1:3s- 38s.

5 Nambudiri DE, Mirchandani IC, Young RC. Two more cases of trazodone related syncope in the eldely. J Geriatric Psychiatry Neurol 1989;2:225.

6 Dordling CM, Mischoulon D, Petersen TJ. Et al. The pharmacologic management of SSRI induced side effects: a survey of psychiatrist. Ann Clin Psychiatry 2002;14:143-147.

20

Venlafaxine

Brand name: Effexor

Mode of action of venlafaxine

1. Venlafaxine is a Serotonin Re-uptake Transporter (SERT) Antagonist: The inhibitory effects of venlafaxine on SERT are *8 times stronger* than its effects on the norepinephrine reuptake transporter (NET).

2. Venlafaxine is a Norepinephrine Re-uptake Transporter (NET) antagonist. The NET, located on the pre-synaptic nerve cell, is responsible for pumping the excess synaptic norepinephrine back into the pre-synaptic nerve cell. Thus the inhibition of NET results in more synaptic norepinephrine. The ability of venlafaxine to inhibit the NET is only evident at venlafaxine doses of 150mg/day and above. On the other hand, it appears that venlafaxine's active metabolite, ODV, has a greater inhibitory effect on NET than the parent drug.

3. Venlafaxine is a Dopamine Reuptake Transporter (DAT) Antagonist: The DAT, located on the pre-synaptic nerve cell, is responsible for pumping the excess synaptic dopamine back into the pre synaptic nerve cell. Therefore, the inhibition of DAT results in more synaptic dopamine. The effect of venlafaxine on DAT occurs in the frontal cortex, and only at very high doses of venlafaxine of 375mg and above.

Note: The inhibition of the SERT, NET and DAT transporters is dose-dependent. At lower doses, venlafaxine will block only SERT. At increasing doses, NET will be inhibited; DAT will only be inhibited at venlafaxine doses of 375mg and above.

Venlafaxine also has an effect on the monoamine reuptake

transporters. This effect is illustrated in Figure 20.1.

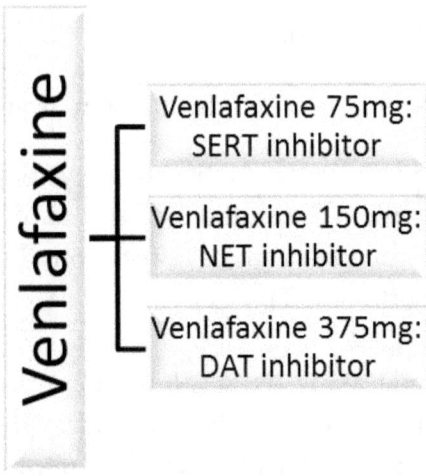

Figure 20.1 Dose-related effects of venlafaxine.

The selective effects of venlafaxine on the anticholinergic, histaminergic and α adrenergic receptors are summarized as follows:

- ✓ **Anticholinergic Ach muscarinic affinity: Low.** Venlafaxine has a low incidence of side effects of dry mouth, constipation, blurred vision and drowsiness.

- ✓ **Histaminergic H1 affinity: Low.** Venlafaxine has a low incidence of side effects of sedation and weight gain.

- ✓ **α 1 adrenergic affinity: Low.** Venlafaxine has a low incidence of side effects of hypotension, dizziness, drowsiness and other cardiovascular effects

Pharmacokinetics of venlafaxine

Venlafaxine has **linear pharmacokinetics,** and it does not inhibit its own metabolism. Each dose increase of venlafaxine may lead to a proportionately greater increase in the venlafaxine plasma levels; thus, the higher the daily dose of venlafaxine, the higher the plasma level will get.

Furthermore, studies suggest that venlafaxine has dose-dependent efficacy, meaning that the higher the daily dose of venlafaxine, the more efficacious it becomes at improving the depressive mood.

In comparison, the venlafaxine XR formulation resulted in a lower Cmax 150ng/ml than the venlafaxine IR formulation (Cmax 225ng/ml). The venlafaxine metabolite ODV has the highest Cmax of 260ng/ml.

Time to peak plasma levels (Tmax.): **1-3 hours** (immediate release), **6 hours** (extended release), **2-6 hours** (active metabolite ODV).

Steady state: Venlafaxine will reach plasma steady state within **3 days** of daily use. Once venlafaxine reaches a plasma steady state, it has less plasma level fluctuations, and it is often associated with a significant reduction in side effects.

Absorption: Venlafaxine is well absorbed by the gastrointestinal system. More than 90% of the oral dose of venlafaxine will be absorbed into the blood circulation. Venlafaxine absorption is not affected by the presence of food or by the stomach pH. The venlafaxine bioavailability is 45%. Venlafaxine has low protein binding properties and less than 35% of the circulating venlafaxine is connected to the plasma protein.

Bioavailability 45%

Protein binding: Venlafaxine has low protein binding properties; less than 35% of the circulating venlafaxine is connected to the plasma protein.

Half-Life: (t1/2): Venlafaxine's elimination half-life is **3-7 hours** (Immediate Release), **15 hours** (extended release); **9-13 hours** (active metabolite ODV). Due to the short half-life of the venlafaxine IR formulation, venlafaxine IR requires twice-a-day dosing. On the other hand, the extended release formulation, which has a longer half-life, can be taken in a single dose. Furthermore, due to its relatively short half-life, abrupt discontinuation of venlafaxine often results in discontinuation syndrome, which can develop even after one missed dose.

Metabolism: Venlafaxine is primarily metabolized by the liver via the enzyme CYP450: **2D6** into an active metabolite: *O-Desmethylvenlafaxine* **(ODV),** which also has antidepressant effects which are as potent as those of the parent drug. The other metabolite of venlafaxine, *N-desmethylvenlafaxine,* has no clinical effects.

Patients that have low CYP 2D6 concentrations in their liver so-called "poor metabolizers", may have increases in their venlafaxine plasma levels and reductions in the ODV plasma levels compared to patients with normal 2D6 enzymes. However, practically speaking, the presence of poor versus extensive venlafaxine metabolizers has no clinical relevance.

It appears that ODV metabolism is not affected by cytochrome 2D6

Patients with liver disease or heavy alcohol abusers can experience a significant decrease in venlafaxine metabolism, which requires a reduction in the dose of venlafaxine by 50%.

P-gp system

Venlafaxine is a *substrate* of the P-gp system as well as **a weak**

inhibitor of P-gp activity. In addition, in vitro, venlafaxine appears to be able to induce the expression of the P-gp.

Elimination: **Urine 87%**. The majority of venlafaxine is eliminated by the urine. Patients with impaired kidneys should use 25% less venlafaxine, while patients who are on haemodialysis should use 50% less venlafaxine.

How supplied

Venlafaxine IR and XR capsules: 37.5 mg, 75mg, 150 mg.

The Extended Release formula requires once a day dosing and has a lower incidence of side effects (particularly, lower incidence of nausea and other gastrointestinal discomfort).

Dose range

- For depression: 75 mg – 225 mg
- For generalized anxiety disorder: 150mg - 225mg once a day.

How to treat

- **For depression:** start venlafaxine with a maximal daily dose of 75 mg, to be increased every 4 days, up to a maximum of 225mg a day. Continue with the higher dose until reaching the desired antidepressant efficacy. In severe cases, the maximum venlafaxine daily dose of 375mg needs to be used. This is attributed to the blocking of NET and DAT which only occur at higher doses of venlafaxine.
- **For generalized anxiety disorder:** start with 75mg a day to be increased weekly up to a maximum of 225mg a day.

When and how to take the medication

Venlafaxine XR should be taken preferably in the morning as a once daily dose (Venlafaxine IR should be taken as a twice a day dose). The patient must avoid crushing or chewing the capsule as it will interfere with the drug absorption.

Clinical indications of venlafaxine

- Major depression
- Generalised anxiety disorder
- Panic disorder
- Social anxiety disorder
- Post traumatic stress disorder
- Premenstrual dysphoric disorder (PMDD)

Major Depressive Disorder (MDD)

Venlafaxine has established its efficacy in the treatment of MDD in both inpatients as well as in outpatients. It appears that venlafaxine has a dose-response effect: The higher the venlafaxine dose, the better the antidepressant effect.

A study conducted in hospitalized patients with major depression and melancholia showed that the patients receiving a venlafaxine dose of 225mg/day had a better antidepressant response than those patients who got fluoxetine or placebo (13). On the other hand, another fixed dose study showed that the antidepressant effects of venlafaxine were smaller at the higher dose of 375mg/day compared to 225mg/day.

Some data suggests that venlafaxine, along with other newer antidepressants such as buprorion and mirtazapine, has a faster and better response rate than the SSRI class (4). In addition, venlafaxine was found to show earlier improvement when compared to the TCA imipramine (7). Moreover, the remission rates of depressed patients treated with SSRIs were only 40% compared to 47% in those patients treated with venlafaxine (1).

According to a meta-analysis of 93 trials (6), it appears that the dual-action SNRI class is more efficacious than the SSRI class for the treatment of major depression.

The efficacy and the remission rates of SNRIs and SSRIs are illustrated in Figure 20.2.

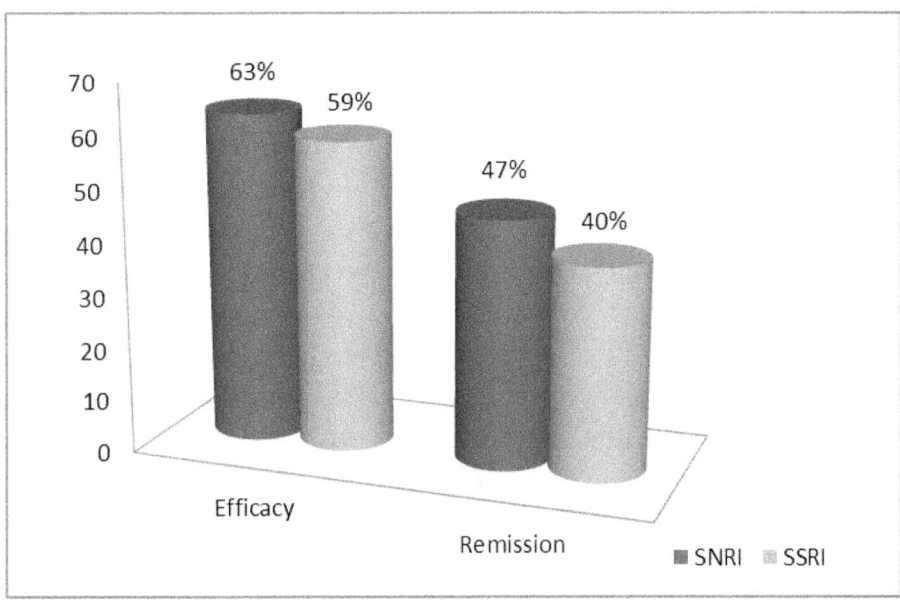

Figure 20.2: 1 Comparison of the efficacy of SNRIs versus SSRIs. Adapted from Papakostas G.I, Thase M.E, Fava M. et al. Are antidepressant drugs that combine serotonergic and noradrenergic mechanisms of action more effective than the selective serotonin reuptake inhibitors in treating MDD? A meta analysis of studies of newer agents. Biological Psychiatry 2007; 62, 1217 – 1227. **2 Comparison of the remission rates of SNRIs versus SSRIs:** Adapted from Nemeroff, CB, Willard, L. Et al: venlafaxine and SSRI: Pooled remission analysis. New research poster presented at the 156th APA annual meeting , San Francisco, CA, May 2003;17-22.

Furthermore, the relapse rate after 6 months and 1 year of treatment with venlafaxine was significantly lower than in those patients who were given placebo.

Potential advantages for the use of venlafaxine

- Venlafaxine was shown to have a dose-response curve with better efficacy for the treatment of major depression at higher doses.
- Desvenlafaxine (the active metabolites of venlafaxine), has a *low affinity for the CYP 2D6 isoenzymes*, which may result in a lower risk of drug interactions.
- Venlafaxine has a low *affinity* for the α-adrenergic, histaminergic and the muscarinic receptors, thereby reducing the unwanted side effects of venlafaxine. This may result in better adherence to treatment.
- Venlafaxine's long-acting formulation may result in fewer side effects, and may facilitate adherence to treatment.

ODV's efficacy for the treatment of major depression

The active metabolite of venlafaxine, desvenlafaxine (ODV) has mechanism of action identical to that of the parent drug venlafaxine, as well as equivalent efficacy for the treatment of major depression (15). Desvenlafaxine (ODV) at doses of 200mg/day and 400mg/day were superior to placebo (14). However, only the 200mg/day of desvenlafaxine dose showed better remission rates than those of placebo.

Generalised Anxiety Disorder (GAD)

Venlafaxine is also highly efficacious for the treatment of GAD.

Venlafaxine appears to be a more effective than placebo even at lower doses of 75mg – 150mg a day, probably due to its effect on the brain levels of serotonin (8,9). In addition, it appears that the antianxiety properties of venlafaxine were apparent as early as the second week of treatment (9), and continued during the 6-month period that was studied.

Social anxiety disorder

Venlafaxine at doses of 150mg a day are effective in controlling the symptoms of social anxiety disorder. In a comparative study of venlafaxine versus paroxetine for the treatment of social anxiety disorder, venlafaxine was shown to be as effective as paroxetine (10).

How to stop the use of venlafaxine

Due to its relatively short half-life, there is a need for a slow tapering of venlafaxine in order to avoid withdrawal symptoms. *It appears that venlafaxine's withdrawal symptoms are more common and more severe compared to other antidepressants.*

Clinical implication: Venlafaxine requires a gradual dose reduction in order to avoid the discontinuation symptoms. The venlafaxine dose should be reduced by 50% every 3-7 days. In the event of getting withdrawal symptoms re instate of the previous dose, and once the discontinuation symptoms disappear, venlafaxine can be reduced in smaller proportions and over a longer period of time.

How long it takes to get an antidepressant effect

In order to get an antidepressant effect, venlafaxine should be used daily for at least 2 – 4 weeks. Although studies did not show increased efficacy above 225mg a day, some patients may benefit from doses of 375mg a day. Like all antidepressants venlafaxine needs time before a substantial mood improvement emerges.

Side effects of venlafaxine

Venlafaxine's side effects are probably related to its ability to increase serotonin and norepinephrine levels in the brain.

Most side effects of venlafaxine develop soon after the initiation of treatment, and are dose- dependent, meaning the higher the dose of venlafaxine, the more prominent the side effects become. In most cases, venlafaxine side effects will gradually subside over time. The most common side effects of venlafaxine are nausea, insomnia, headache, sweating and dizziness.

The most common side effects with the use of venlafaxine are as follows:

The nervous system

Venlafaxine is less activating compared to the SSRIs. The sedating effects of venlafaxine appear to be equivalent to SSRIs, but to a lesser degree than TCAs.

- Insomnia
- Nervousness
- Anxiety
- Restless leg syndrome
- Muscle spasm
- Tremor
- Hot flushes
- Headache
- Dizziness
- Blurred vision
- Seizures (rare, mainly associated with treatment discontinuation)

- Increased sweating
- Fatigue
- Somnolence
- Sedation
- Rash
- Hypertension

Cardiac

Increased blood pressure affects 2%-6% of the patients treated with venlafaxine, and it appears to be dose-related. Thus up to 12% of patients treated with venlafaxine at a mean dose of 350mg/day may develop hypertension.

Gastro intestinal

Venlafaxine often results in GI side effects, which can develop within 30 minutes of drug ingestion. It appears that the gastro intestinal side effects of venlafaxine are more likely the result of the direct effect of venlafaxine on the intestinal mucosa than its effects on the CNS or plasma concentration. Weight gain is a troublesome side effect associated with venlafaxine. Weight gain will develop slowly and can affect up to 16% of treated patients, and is comparable to weight gain with SSRIs.

- Decreased appetite
- Nausea
- Weight gain although weight loss is possible.
- Vomiting
- Dry mouth
- Diarrhea
- Constipation
- Gastritis

Sexual

The sexual-related side effects of venlafaxine will develop soon after the commencement of treatment and are relatively high but are comparable to those of SSRIs. Up to 30% of patients treated with venlafaxine can develop sexual impairments. The sexual side effects of venlafaxine are probably related to its effects on serotonin, and are more prominent in males than in females. Furthermore, it appears that the risk of sexual dysfunction is correlated with age and with higher venlafaxine doses.

- Decreased sex drive
- Delayed ejaculation
- Impotence
- Abnormal orgasm

Suicide

The FDA requires all antidepressants to carry a black box warning stating that antidepressants may increase the risk of suicide in persons under the age of 25 years. This warning is based on data suggesting that suicidal ideations and behavior has a 2-fold increase in children and in adolescents, and a 1.5 – fold increase in the 18 – 24 age group.

Practical management of venlafaxine side effects

As a general rule, venlafaxine side effects are dose- dependent: the higher the dose of venlafaxine, the worse the side effect. Lowering the dose of venlafaxine is often associated with the resolution of side effects. In the event of persistent and debilitating side effects which continue despite dose reduction switching to another antidepressant class may result in their resolution. However, there are some side effects which can be associated with venlafaxine, which merit urgent and immediate attention.

Venlafaxine side effects that need immediate attention

- Confusion
- Excitation
- Onset of seizure
- Yellow skin / eyes
- Severe allergic reaction
- Irregular heart beat
- Hypertension
- Induction of manic or hypomanic episode
- Activation of suicidal ideation and behaviour

Venlafaxine discontinuation reaction

The sudden discontinuation of venlafaxine can be associated with a discontinuation reaction, which is self-limiting. The withdrawal symptoms of venlafaxine can develop within 8 – 16 hours of its discontinuation and can last up to 8 days. The most common symptoms of venlafaxine discontinuation reaction are:

- Irritability
- Agitation
- Dizziness
- Nausea
- Electric shock sensations
- Diarrhea
- Muscle cramps
- Anxiety
- Confusion
- Nightmares
- Headache
- Lethargy
- Insomnia
- Seizures
- Dysphoric mood

A gradual down-titration of venlafaxine often reduces the risk of developing a discontinuation reaction.

Safety profile of venlafaxine

Use in pregnancy: Risk category C

Venlafaxine is not evidently teratogenic.

However, the use of venlafaxine during the first trimester as well as throughout the pregnancy is not recommended. One study released in Canada suggests that venlafaxine use during pregnancy can double the risk of miscarriage.

Use during lactation

Venlafaxine is secreted in the breast milk in considerable quantities. Furthermore, breast-fed infants of mothers treated with venlafaxine had detectable serum venlafaxine levels.

Due to its unknown effects on the newborn's normal growth and development, breast feeding should be avoided in women who are using venlafaxine.

Special considerations with the use of venlafaxine

- **Narrow-angle glaucoma**: Venlafaxine can increase eye pressure due to its ability to potentiate the effects of norepinephrine (NE). Venlafaxine should be avoided in patients having un-controlled narrow-angle glaucoma.
- **Hypertension**: The Venlafaxine potentiating effects on norepinephrine (NE) can lead to increased heart rates and blood pressure. It appears that 2 – 6% of patients who are getting venlafaxine will experience an increased diastolic blood pressure; this appears to be dose-dependent.
- **PPHN**: Venlafaxine use was associated with persistent pulmonary hypertension (PPHN).

- **ECG**: Venlafaxine has no clinical effects on the ECG profile and on the QTc interval. It has been shown to be safe for the treatment of depression in patients with myocardial infarction and angina. However, in animal models, venlafaxine appears to be able to block the myocardial sodium channels; this has an unclear clinical implication.
- **Overdose fatalities**: There are several reports of fatal cardiotoxicity following venlafaxine overdose. Furthermore, overdose with venlafaxine may result in higher mortality rates than overdose with SSRIs (11).
- **Rhabdomyolysis**: There are several reports of rhabdomyolysis with the use of venlafaxine (12).
- **REM sleep**: Venlafaxine can supress REM sleep.
- **Bruxism**: Venlafaxine may cause bruxism.
- **Abnormal bleeding**: Venlafaxine may lead to abnormal bleeding and bruising. Concomitant use of warfarin, NSAIDs and aspirin may add to this risk.
- **Urinary hesitancy**: Venlafaxine's ability to potentiate norepinephrine (NE) can increase urethral resistance, which might lead to urinary hesitancy.
- **Prostatic hypertrophy**: Venlafaxine should be used with caution in patients with prostatic hypertrophy due to possible urinary hesitancy and urinary retention.

Venlafaxine drug interactions

Follows a list of venlafaxine's drug interactions
- **Warfarin:** The concomitant use may displace warfarine from its protein which may result in increased INR, which might lead to a possible risk of bleeding.
- **Fluvoxamine:** The concomitant use may increase venlafaxine plasma levels with a possible increase in blood pressure and anticholinergic effects which

include dry mouth, constipation, blurred vision and urinary retention.
- **Bupropion:** The concomitant use may cause a 3-fold increase in venlafaxine plasma levels.
- **Cimetidine & other H2 antagonists:** The concomitant use may increase venlafaxine plasma levels by 60%.
- **MAOI:** The concomitant use may cause CNS toxicity - serotonin syndrome. Wait 21 days after the MAOI was stopped before initiating treatment with venlafaxine. After discontinuing venlafaxine, wait 7 days before starting a MAOI.
- **Zolpidem:** The concomitant use may cause delirium.
- **Beta Blokers**: The concomitant use may increase venlafaxine plasma level due to the competition for CYP 2D6 liver enzyme.
- **Tramadol:** The concomitant use may increase the risk of seizures.

Warnings for venlafaxine

Pregnancy: Risk category C. Try to avoid use during pregnancy or breastfeeding. Assessment of the risks versus benefits must be discussed with the patient.

> **Suicide in children & young adults**: Venlafaxine may cause an increase in suicidal risk in young adults, and it carries a black box warning. Venlafaxine may cause a **5-fold increase** in suicidal ideations and suicidal behaviour in patients under 25 years of age. On the other hand, FDA analysis of suicide risk among adults using venlafaxine showed no significant difference from fluoxetine or placebo. Venlafaxine is contra indicated in children, adolescents and young adults due to the possible risk of suicide.

- **Serotonin syndrome:** Venlafaxine may cause serotonin syndrome. Serotonin syndrome symptoms include agitation, dizziness, hallucinations, delirium, seizures and coma along with autonomic instability, which includes tachycardia, fluctuating blood pressure, flushing, hyperthermia, tremor, muscular rigidity, myoclonus, hyperreflexia, and incoordination. The concomitant use of venlafaxine with a MAOI may precipitate serotonin syndrome which may be fatal.
- **MAOI:** Venlafaxine requires a *1 week washout period* before starting treatment with a MAOI. After a MAOI is stopped a *3- week washout period* is required before starting venlafaxine.
- **Renal impairment:** Venlafaxine requires a lower dose in mild to moderate renal impairment.
- **Liver insufficiency:** Venlafaxine should be avoided in patients with liver insufficiency.
- **Alcohol abuse:** Venlafaxine is not recommended in patients abusing alcohol, due to the effects on the liver.
- **Mania & hypomania:** Venlafaxine may trigger mania in predisposed patients. It should be used cautiously in patients with a history of bipolar mood disorder.
- **Elderly:** Venlafaxine needs a lower dose when it is used in the elderly.

Overdose with venlafaxine

Overdose with venlafaxine can be lethal. Data from the U.K suggests that venlafaxine overdose carries a higher rate of lethality when compared with SSRI overdose. Death was reported following ingestion of very large doses of venlafaxine. Venlafaxine plasma levels within the range of 10 -90 mg/L was associated with fatalities. In addition, the concomitant use of venlafaxine with alcohol and/ or with other central nervous depressants such as painkillers or benzo-diazepines may result in death caused by respiratory depression.

General symptom of venlafaxine overdose

Initially, the patient might feel extremely tired and lethargic. The pulse will slow down, and the breathing frequency will decrease.

As the level of intoxication increases, the level of consciousness will decrease, and the patient will become unresponsive to external stimulations. The reflexes will disappear, and the breathing will get shallow. The patient's pulse and blood pressure will drop until cardiovascular system collapse.

The most common symptoms of venlafaxine overdose are

- vomiting
- over-sedation/ agitation
- seizures
- abnormal heart rhythm-tachycardia
- hypertension

What to do in the case of venlafaxine overdose

In general, there is no antidote for venlafaxine overdose. Management is mainly supportive, aimed at maintaining respiration, pulse and blood pressure. In the event of a recent overdose with venlafaxine, a stomach washout with activated charcoal might help in the elimination of the un-absorbed drug and is done with a large bore oro-gastric tube with appropriate airway protection. The aim of the stomach lavage is to get rid of the drug leftovers.

In some ER departments, ipecac is also used in order to induce vomiting of the ingested toxin, however **induction of emesis is not recommended in semi-comatose and comatose patients.**

Due to the large volume of distribution of venlafaxine, forced diuresis, dialysis hemo-perfusion and exchange transfusion are unlikely to be effective.

Keeping open the patient's airway is compulsory, especially in semi - comatose individuals. The patient should be placed on his side in order to prevent aspiration of the vomitus back to the lungs. Suffocation due to vomit is the leading cause of death in venlafaxine overdose. Blood pressure and heart rate monitoring is very important. Fluid intake should be monitored with intravenous infusion of saline, and urinary output should also be carefully monitored. In most cases, venlafaxine overdose, requires hospitalization of the patient for at least 24 hours for intense observation.

Venlafaxine references.

1. Nemeroff, CB, Willard, L. Et al: venlafaxine and SSRI: Pooled remission analysis. New research poster presented at the 156th APA annual meeting , San Francisco, CA, May2003; 17-22.

2 Schmitt A.B, Bauer, M. et al. Differential effects of venlafaxine in the treatment of MDD according to baseline severity. European Archives of Psychiatry and Clinical Neuroscience, 2009;259, 329 – 339.

3 Kornstein, S.G, Mao, .Y et al. Escitalopram versus SNRI antidepressants in the acute treatment of major depressive disorder. CNS Spectrums, 2009;14(6), 326-333.

4 Davidson J.R, Meoni P. et al,. Archieving remission with venlafaxine and fluoxetine in major depression: its relationship to anxiety symptoms. Depression and anxiety, 2002;16(1), 4-13.

5 Thase, M.E, Entsuah, et al. Relative antidepressant efficacy of venlafaxine and SSRIs: sex- age interaction. Journal of woman Health, 2005;14, 6009-616.

6 Papakostas G.I, Thase M.E, Fava M. et al. Are antidepressant drugs that combine serotonergic and noradrenergic mechanisms of action more effective than the selective serotonin reuptake inhibitors in treating MDD? A meta analysis of studies of newer agents. Biological Psychiatry 2007;62, 1217 - 1227.

7 Benkert,O., Grunder, G, Wetzel, H et al. A randomized double blind comparison of a rapid escalating dose of venlafaxine and imipramine in inpatients with MDD and melancholia. Journal of Psychiatric Research, 1996;30(6), 441 - 451.

8 Rickels K., Pollack M., Sheehan D. et al. Efficacy of XR venlafaxine in non - depressed outpatients with GAD. Am. J. Psychiatry 2000;157: 968 - 974.

9 Allgulander C, Hackett D, Salinas E et al. Venlafaxine ER in the treatment of GAD: twenty - four week placebo - controlled dose - ranging study. Br J. Psychiatry 2001;179:15-22.

10 Allgulander C., Mangano R, Zhang J, et al Efficacy of venlafaxine ER in patients with SAD. A double blind, placebo - controlled , parallel group comparison with Paroxetine. Human Psychopharmacology 2004;19: 387 - 396.

11 Flanagan, R.J,. Fatal toxicity of drugs used in psychiatry. Human Psychopharmacology, 2008;23 (Supp. 1), 43 - 51.

12 Wilson A. D, Howell, C, & Waring, W. Venlafaxine ingestion is associated with rhabdomyolysis in adults: A case serie. J. of Toxicological Sciences, 2007;32 (1), 97 - 101.

13 Clerc GE, Ruimy P, Verdeau- Pailes J. A double blind comparison of venlafaxine and fluoxetine in patients hospitalized for MDD and melancholia. Int. Clin. Psychopharmacol. 1994; 9:139-143.

14 Septien- Velez L, Pitroski B., Padmanahan SK et al, . A randomized double blind, placebo controlled trial of desvenlafaxine succinate in the treatment of MDD. Int. Clin. Psychopharmacol. 2007;22:338-347.

15 Lieberman, D.Z, Montgomery, SA, Tourian, K et al. A pooled analysis of two placebo – controlled trials of desvenlafaxine in major depressive disorder. Int. Clin. Psychopharmacol.2008; 23 (4), 188 – 197.

21

Vilazodone

Brand name:

Viibryd

Vilazodone's Mode of Action

1. Vilazodone is a Serotonin Reuptake Transporter (SERT) antagonist: The inhibition of the SERT located on the presynaptic neurons by vilazodone results in increased serotonin synaptic levels..

2. Vilazodone is a partial agonist of 5-HT1A receptors: The inhibition of the postsynaptic 5-HT1A receptors will activate the release of dopamine from the dopaminergic nerve cells.

Vilazodone Pharmacokinetics

Vilazodone has **linear pharmacokinetics which are dose-dependent.** Thus, any dose increase leads to a proportional increase in the drug plasma levels.

Peak plasma levels (Tmax): 4-5 hours. Vilazodone's side effects tend to emerge at the peak of its plasma level. A single dose of vilazodone may result in emerging side effects 4 hours after drug ingestion.

Absorption: Vilazodone is well absorbed by the gastrointestinal system. The administration of vilazodone with food will *increase* it oral bioavailability by 160% and its AUC by 85%. However, if vomiting occurs within 7 hours of ingestion, vilazodone's absorption is decreased by 25%.

Elimination half-life (t ½): 25 hours for the parent drug.

Bioavailability: 72%

Protein binding: 96-99%. Vilazodone is highly protein bound. Up to 99% of the circulating vilazodone is attached to plasma albumin.

Steady state: Vilazodone will reach a steady state concentration within **3 days** of regular use.

Metabolism: Vilazodone is primarily metabolised by the liver via the enzyme CYP450: **3A4**. Only 1% of vilazodone is excreted in the urine as unchanged vilazodone.

In vitro studies with human microsomes and human hepatocytes showed that vilazodone is unlikely to inhibit or induce the metabolism of other CYP enzymes. However, strong inhibitors of the CYP 3A4 enzyme (such as ketoconazole) can reduce vilazodone metabolism, which may result in increased vilazodone plasma levels.

Similarly, CYP 3A4 inducers may decrease vilazodone plasma concentrations.

The P-gp System

The effects of vilazodone on the P-gp system are still unknown.

Elimination: **Urine >80%.** The presence of mild to moderate renal impairment as well as mild to moderate liver impairment does not affect the vilazodone clearance.

How supplied

- Tablets 10mg, 20mg, and 40mg.

Dose range

10mg - 40mg a day for depression

How to treat

- **For Depression:** Start with vilazodone 10mg a day, ingested preferably with food, for seven days, followed by an increase to 20mg for an additional seven days, and then increase to 40mg a day. The maximum dose should be lowered to a 20mg a day when it is co- administered with CYP 3A4 inhibitors, such as the antifungal ketoconazole, protease inhibitors, macrolides and verapamil.

When and how to take medication

Preferably take vilazodone at bedtime to avoid over-sedation. In general, use the principle "start low and go slow" as patients can experience over-sedation the following day at the beginning of the treatment.

Vilazodone clinical indications

- Major depression

Major Depressiive Disorder (MDD)

The efficacy of vilazodone in the treatment of depression was established in two pivotal 8-week randomized double-blind placebo-controlled trials.

The first pivotal trial (3) involved 410 outpatients who were randomly assigned to vilazodone or placebo.

By the end of the study, the vilazodone treated patients showed a statistically significant improvement on the primary efficacy measure which was the Montgomery- Asberg Depression Rating Scale (MADRAS). They also had a statistically significant improvement on the secondary efficacy measures which were the Hamilton Rating Scale for Depression (HAMD-17) and the Clinical Global Impression Improvement scale (CGI-I). The rates of discontinuation due to adverse events were 5.1% for vilazodone and 1.7% for placebo. The results of this study are illustrated in Figure 21.1

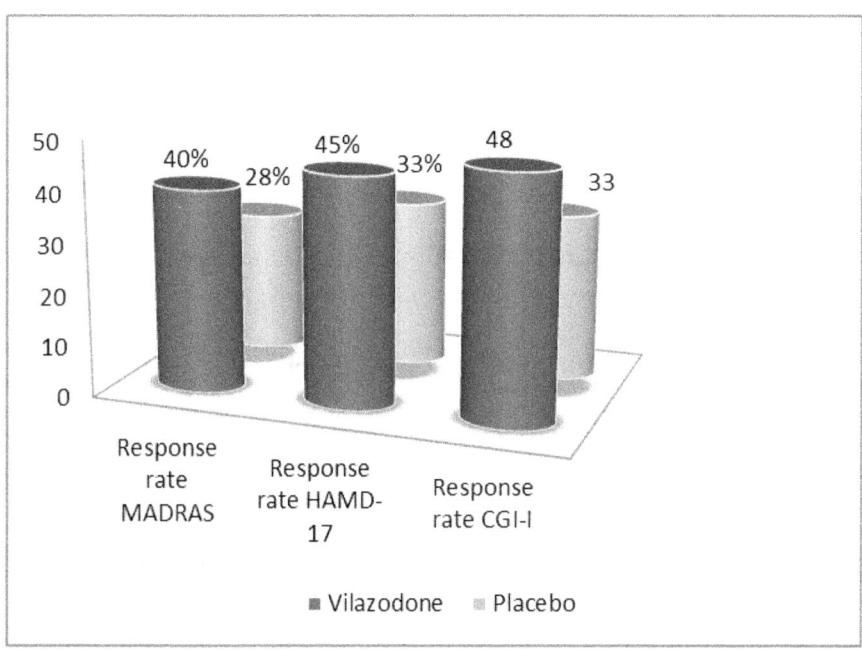

Figure 21.1 Vilazodone and Placebo response rates in the treatment of MDD using the MADRAS, HAMD-17 and CGI-I scoring systems. Adapted from Rickels response study: Rickels K, Athanaasiou M, Robinson DS et al. Evidence for efficacy and tolerability of vilazodone in the treatment of MDD; a randomized, double-blind,placebo-controlled trial. J Clin Psychiatry. 2009;70(3);326-333

How to stop vilazodone

It is highly recommended to taper vilazodone slowly in order to minimize the emergence of withdrawal symptoms, which usually develop within the first 2 weeks of treatment cessation. A 50% dose reduction every third day is recommended. In the event of the patient developing withdrawal symptoms, re-instate the previous dose, and once the symptoms disappear, start reducing the vilazodone dose in a smaller proportions and over a longer period of time.

How long it takes to get an antidepressant effect

Like all antidepressants, vilazodone needs at least 7 – 28 days before a substantial mood improvement emerges.

Vilazodone side effects

Most side effects of vilazodone are probably related to its ability to increase serotonin in the brain. Vilazodone's side effects are usually dose-related and often develop soon after the initiation of treatment, and subside with time. The most common side effects of vilazodone are diarrhea, nausea and headache.

Nervous system

- dizziness
- somnolence
- paresthesias
- tremor
- insomnia
- abnormal dreams
- restlessness
- fatigue
- feeling jittery
- headache and worsening of migraine

- *seizures.*

Gastro intestinal

The gastro intestinal side effects can develop within 30 minutes of drug ingestion, and they are more likely the result of the effects of vilazodone on the serotonin uptake.

- Nausea
- Diarrhea
- Dry mouth
- Vomiting
- Dyspepsia
- Flatulance
- Gastroenteritis
- Heartburn
- Increased appetite

Sexual

The incidence of sexual side effects with vilazodone are relatively low.

- decreased libido
- erectile dysfunction
- abnormal orgasm
- delayed ejaculation

Vilazodone side effects that need immediate attention

- Confusion
- Excitation
- Onset of seizure
- Yellow skin / eyes
- Severe allergic reaction
- Irregular heart beat

- Hypotension
- Induction of manic or hypomanic episode
- Activation of suicidal ideation and behaviour especially in children and adolescents

Physical and psychological dependence

Vilazodone did not show any tendencies for drug seeking behavior. However, patients with a history of drug abuse should be closely monitored for signs of vilazodone misuse or abuse, which includes drug seeking behavior, development of tolerance and unsolicited dose increases.

Discontinuation reaction of vilazodone

Sudden discontinuation of vilazodone may be associated with a discontinuation reaction. The discontinuation symptoms are usually self-limiting. The most common symptoms of discontinuation reaction are:

- irritability
- agitation
- dizziness
- anxiety
- confusion
- headache
- lethargy
- insomnia
- seizures
- dysphoric mood
- fever
- fatigue
- sweating
- myalgia (muscle pain)
- electric shock sensation

A slow down-titration of vilazodone may reduces the risk of having the discontinuation reaction.

Suicide

The FDA requires all antidepressants to carry a black box warning stating that antidepressants may increase the risk of suicide in persons under the age of 25 years. This warning is based on data suggesting that suicidale ideations and behavior has a 2-fold increase in children and in adolescents, and a 1.5 – fold increase in the 18 – 24 age group.

Safety profile of vilazodone

Use in pregnancy: Risk category C

There are no adequate well controlled studies of vilazodone in pregnant women.

Vilazodone was not teratogenic in rats or rabbits during the period of organogenesis at oral doses up to 48 times the maximum recommended human dose (MRHD).

Fetal body weight was reduced and skeletal ossification was delayed in both rats and rabbits exposed to high doses of vilazodone. Furthermore, the administration of vilazodone to pregnant rats at a dose of 30 times the MRHD there was an increase in early postnatal pup mortality, delayed maturation and decreased fertility in adulthood.

In addition, the use of vilazodone, like with all antidepressants, in the last trimester of pregnancy was associated with higher incidence of respiratory distress and pulmonary hypertension, cyanosis, apnea, seizures, temperature instability vomiting, hypoglycemia, hypotonia, hyperreflexia, tremor, irritability, constant crying and jitteriness, which required prolonged hospitalization, tube feeding and respiratory support.

The risk of the newborn to develop Persistent Pulmonary Hypertension of the Newborns (PPHN) is substantially higher comaperd to pregnant woman not on antidepressants. PPHN is associated with substantial neonatal morbidity and mortality.

Thus, the use of vilazodone during the first trimester as well as throughout the pregnancy is not recommended.

Use during lactation

Vilazodone is secreted in the human breast milk. Due to its unknown effects on the newborn's normal growth and development breast feeding should be avoided.

Carcinogenesis

There is no evidence of carcinogenesis, teratogenicity, mutagenicity or impaired fertility with vilazodone use.

Avoid using vilazodone in the following cases

- **Patients with known allergy to vilazodone**
- **Patients with a history of seizure**

Vilazodone's drug interactions

Follows a list of vilazodone's drug interactions

- **Tramadol**: The concomitant use may increase the risk of seizure.
- **Warfarin**: The concomitant use may cause an increase in PT.
- **Carbamazepine**: The concomitant use may decrease vilazodone plasma levels.
- **Ketoconazole**: The concomitant use may increase vilazodone plasma levels.

- **MAOI:** The concomitant use may cause Serotonin syndrome. Patients must wait 21 days after the MAOI was stopped before initiating treatment with vilazodone. Wait 5-7 days after discontinuing vilazodone before starting a MAOI.
- **Grapefruit Juice:** The concomitant use may decrease vilazodone metabolism due to inhibition of the P450 **3A4**.
- **Tamoxifen:** The concomitant use may decrease vilazodone plasma levels.
- **Triptans:** The concomitant use may cause serotonin syndrome.
- **Ketoconazole:** The concomitant use may increase vilazodone plasma levels.
- **Verapamil:** The concomitant use may increase vilazodone plasma levels.

Warning for vilazodone

- **Pregnancy: Risk category C.** Try to avoid use during pregnancy or breast feeding. Assessment of the risks versus benefits must be discussed with the patient.
- **Seizure risk.** Vilazodone was not associated with increased seizure activity. However, patients with a history of seizure require caution when using vilazodone, as well as patients with an increased predisposition to have seizures, such as brain damage, as well as alcohol abusers.
- **Vilazodone may cause an increase in suicidal risk in young adults.** The use of antidepressants in this population must balance the risk of suicide with the clinical need. Careful monitoring of the patients clinical worsening is necessary. Evaluation for suicidality should also involve the family and all other caregivers.

- **Activation of hypomania or mania** may occur in vilazodone-treated bipolar patients. As vilazodone may trigger mania in predisposed patients, it should be used cautiously in patients with a history of bipolar mood disorder
- **Serotonin syndrome** may develop with vilazodone use. Serotonin syndrome symptoms may include agitation, dizziness, hallucinations, delirium, seizures and coma along with autonomic instability, which includes tachycardia, fluctuating blood pressure, flushing, hyperthermia, tremor, muscular rigidity, myoclonus, hyperreflexia and incoordination. The concomitant use of vilazodone with MAOIs, triptans, TCAs, lithium, fentanyl, tramadol, tryptophan, buspirone and St. John's Wort may precipitate serotonin syndrome.
- **Renal impairment**: Vilazodone does not require a lower dose in mild to moderate renal impairment.
- **Liver impairment**: Vilazodone does not require lower dose in patients with liver impairment..
- **Alcohol:** Vilazodone is not recommended in patients abusing alcohol.
- **Withdrawal reaction**. Vilazodone use may result in a withdrawal reaction, prevention of which requires a slow reduction of vilazodone dose. The onset of withdrawal symptoms is attributed to vilazodone's relatively short half-life. The withdrawal symptoms of vilazodone can develop as early as the second day of the drug's sudden discontinuation and may persist for several days. The most common withdrawal symptoms are nausea, dizziness, insomnia, anxiety, tension and headache.
- **MAOI:** Vilazodone's combined use with a MAOI may be fatal. Vilazodone requires **7 day** washout period before starting with a MAOI. A **3 week** washout period is needed

after the MAOI was stopped before starting with vilazodone.
- ➢ **Weight**: Vilazodone was not associated with weight gain.
- ➢ **Abnormal bleeding:** The use of vilazodone and SSRIs may be associated with increased risk of bleeding. The concomitant use of aspirin, NSAIDs and warfarin may add to this risk. Bleeding has ranged from ecchymosis, hematoma, epistaxis and petechiae to life-threatening hemorrhage.
- ➢ **Hyponatremias**: No cases of hyponatremia were reported with the use of vilazodone.

Vilazodone overdose

There is limited clinical experience regarding vilazodone overdose. There are only several overdose cases with vilazodone, all of which resulted in a full recovery.

The effects of vilazodone overdose are also dependent on whether it was ingested alone or as a combination with other drugs and or with alcohol. As a general rule, the bigger the amount of vilazodone ingested, the worse the toxic effects and the higher the possibility for lethal results.

General symptoms of vilazodone overdose

Initially, the patient might feel extremely tired and lethargic. The pulse will slow down, and the breathing frequency will decrease. As the level of intoxication increases, the level of consciousness will decrease, and the patient will become unresponsive to external stimulations. The reflexes will disappear, and the breathing will get shallow. The patients pulse and blood pressure will drop until cardiovascular system collapse.

Vilazodone was not lethal in mono therapy overdose.

The concomitant use of vilazodone with alcohol and with other central nervous depressants such as painkillers or benzodiazepines may result in death caused by respiratory depression. The possible fatalities are often the result of cardio-respiratory arrest and the metabolic acidosis and hypoxia which are associated with status epilepticus.

Symptoms of vilazodone over dose are

- Lethargy
- Restlessness
- Hallucinations
- Disorientation
- Serotonin syndrome

What to do in the case of overdose

In general, there is no antidote for vilazodone overdose. Management is mainly supportive, aimed at maintaining respiration, pulse and blood pressure. In the event of a recent overdose with vilazodone, a stomach washout with activated charcoal might help in the elimination of the un-absorbed drug and is done with a large bore oro-gastric tube with appropriate airway protection. The aim of the stomach lavage is to get rid of the drug leftovers.

In some ER departments, ipecac is also used in order to induce vomiting of the ingested toxin, however **induction of emesis is not recommended in semi-comatose and comatose patients**. Due to the large volume of distribution of vilazodone, forced diuresis, dialysis hemo-perfusion and exchange transfusion are unlikely to be effective. Keeping open the patient's airway is compulsory, especially in semi - comatose individuals. The patient should be placed on his side in order to prevent aspiration of the vomitus back to the lungs. Suffocation due to vomit is the leading cause of death in vilazodone overdose. Blood pressure and heart rate monitoring is very important. Fluid intake should be monitored with intra-venous infusion of saline, and urinary output should also be carefully monitored. In most cases, vilazodone overdose, requires hospitalization of the patient for at least 24 hours for intense observation.

Vilazodone references

1 Akamine, Yumiko,Yasui-Furukori et al. Psychotropic drug – drug interactions involving P-gp. Nov 2012 Vol 26 issue 11- 959 – 973

2 Weiss j, Dormann SM, Martin- Facklam et al. Inhibition of P-gp by newer antidepressants. J. Pharmacol Exp Ther. Apr 2003; 305(1):197-204.

3 Rickels K, Athanaasiou M, Robinson DS et al. Evidence for efficacy and tolerability of vilazodone in the treatment of MDD; a randomized, double-blind,placebo-controlled trial. J Clin Psychiatry. 2009;70(3);326-333.

22

Vortioxetine

Brand name: Brintellix

Vortioxetine's Mode of Action

1. Vortioxetine is a Serotonin Reuptake Transporter (SERT) antagonist: The inhibition of the SERT located on the presynaptic neurons by vortioxetine results in increased serotonin synaptic levels..

2. Vortioxetine is a partial near full agonist of the 5-HT1A receptors:

The activation of the postsynaptic 5-HT1A receptors will activate the release of dopamine from the dopaminergic nerve cells which may enhance their antianxiety, cognitive and antidepressant effects.

3 Vortioxetine is a 5-HT3A antagonist:

The inhibitory effects of vortioxetine on the 5-HT3A post synaptic receptors may inhibit the actions of the inhibitory interneurons which may reduce nausea and vomiting.

4 Vortioxetine is a 5-HT7 antagonist

The inhibitory effects of vortioxetine on the 5-HT7 receptors may be involved with the regulation of the circadian rhythms, thus improving sleep and emotions.

5 Vortioxetine is a 5-HT1B partial agonist

6 Vortioxetine is a 5-HT1D receptor antagonist

Vortioxetine Pharmacokinetics

Vortioxetine has **linear pharmacokinetics which are dose-dependent.** Thus, any dose increase leads to a proportional increase in the drug plasma levels.

Peak plasma levels (Tmax): 7-11 hours. Vortioxetine's side effects tend to emerge at the peak of its plasma level. A single dose of vortioxetine may result in emerging side effects 7 hours after drug ingestion.

Absorption: Vortioxetine is well absorbed by the gastrointestinal system.

Elimination half- life (t ½): 66 hours for the parent drug.

Bioavailability: 75%

Protein binding: 98%. Vortioxetine is highly protein bound. Up to 98% of the circulating vortioxetine is attached to plasma albumin.

Steady state: Vortioxetine will reach a steady state concentration within **2 weeks** of regular use.

Metabolism: Vortioxetine is primarily metabolised by the liver via the enzyme CYP450: **2D6.** In addition, vortioxetine is also metabolized by CYP 3A4/4, CYP 2C19, CYP 2C9, CYP 2A6 and CYP 2C8 and CYP 2B6.

2D6 is the primary enzyme catalyzing the metabolism of vortioxetine to its pharmacological inactive, carboxylic acid metabolite.

Poor metabolizers of 2D6 may have twice the vortioxetine plasma concentration of extensive metabolizers.

Excretion: 59% in urine, 26% in Feces.

The presence of hepatic or renal impairment did not affect the clearance of vortioxetine.

The P-gp System

The effects of vortioxetine on the P-gp system are still unknown.

How supplied

- Tablets: 5mg, 10mg, 15mg, 20mg.

Dose range

10mg - 20mg a day for depression

How to treat

- **For Depression:** Start with vortioxetine 10mg a day, ingested preferably with food, for seven days, followed by an increase up to a maximum of 20mg a day.

When and how to take medication

Preferably take vortioxetine once a day. In general, use the principle "start low and go slow" as patients can experience side effects at the beginning of the treatment.

Vortioxetine clinical indications

- Major depression

Major Depressive Disorder (MDD)

The efficacy of vortioxetine in the treatment of depression was established in six pivotal 8-weeks randomized, double-blind placebo-controlled trials.

Early study published in the Int Clin Psychopharmacology May 2014 vortioxetine efficacy and safety at doses of 15mg and 20mg a day were assessed in a randomized, double blind, placebo controlled, duloxetine- referenced study in the acute treatment of adult patients with major depressive disorder.

The study included 608 patients randomly assigned to vortioxetine 15mg, 20mg, duloxetine 60mg or placebo. The primary efficacy endpoint was change from baseline in MADRAS total score at week 8. Both vortioxetine doses were statistically significantly superior to placebo. Duloxetine also separated from placebo, validating the study

In another randomized, placebo controlled FDA submission, doses of vortioxetine 5mg and 10mg were compared to placebo with MADRAS rating scale as the primary outcome measure. The mean change in MADRAS at the end of the 8 week study in vortioxetine 5mg and 10mg were -15.4 and -16.2 respectively compared to -11.3 in the placebo group.

How to stop vortioxetine

It is highly recommended to taper vortioxetine slowly in order to minimize the emergence of withdrawal symptoms, which usually develop within the first week of treatment cessation. A 50% dose reduction every third day is recommended. In the event of the patient developing withdrawal symptoms, re-instate the previous dose, and once the symptoms disappear, start reducing the vortioxetine dose in a smaller proportions and over a longer period of time.

How long it takes to get an antidepressant effect

Like all antidepressants, vortioxetine needs at least 7 – 28 days before a substantial mood improvement emerges.

Vortioxetine side effects

Most side effects of vortioxetine are probably related to its ability to increase serotonin in the brain. Vortioxetine's side effects are usually dose-related and often develop soon after the initiation of treatment, and subside with time. The most common side effects of vortioxetine are diarrhea, nausea and dry mouth.

Nervous system (incidence not known)

- dizziness
- abnormal dreams
- agitation
- confusion
- convulsion
- headache

Gastro intestinal

Nausea was the most commonly observed adverse reaction. Nausea most commonly occurred in the first week of treatment in up to 20% of the treated patients.

- nausea
- diarrhea
- dry mouth
- vomiting
- constipation
- flatulance

Sexual

The incidence of sexual side effects with vortioxetine are relatively low 3%-5%.

- decreased libido
- erectile dysfunction

- abnormal orgasm
- delayed ejaculation

Vortioxetine side effects that need immediate attention

- Confusion
- Excitation
- Onset of seizure
- Yellow skin / eyes
- Severe allergic reaction
- Irregular heart beat
- Hypotension
- Induction of manic or hypomanic episode
- Activation of suicidal ideation and behaviour especially in children and adolescents

Physical and psychological dependence

Vortioxetine effects on drug seeking behavior is unknown. However, patients with a history of drug abuse should be closely monitored for signs of vortioxetine misuse or abuse, which includes drug seeking behavior, development of tolerance and unsolicited dose increases.

Discontinuation reaction of vortioxetine

Sudden discontinuation of vortioxetine at a daily dose of 15-20mg/day may experience discontinuation reaction. The discontinuation symptoms are usually self-limiting. The most common symptoms of discontinuation reaction are:

- headache
- anger
- muscle tension
- mood swings
- dizziness

- runny nose

A slow down-titration of vortioxetine may reduce the risk of having the discontinuation reaction.

Suicide

The FDA requires all antidepressants to carry a black box warning stating that antidepressants may increase the risk of suicide in persons under the age of 25 years. This warning is based on data suggesting that suicide ideations and behavior has a 2-fold increase in children and in adolescents, and a 1.5 – fold increase in the 18 – 24 age group.

Safety profile of vortioxetine

Use in pregnancy: Risk category C

There are no adequate well controlled studies of vortioxetine in pregnant women.

Vortioxetine caused developmental delays in pregnant rats at doses 15 times the maximum recommended human dose (MRHD). There was no teratogenic effects in in rats or rabbits during the period of organogenesis at doses up to 77 times the maximum recommended human dose (MRHD). The incidence of malformations in human pregnancies has not been established.

Vortioxetine should be used during pregnancy only if the potential benefit outweigh the potential risk to the fetus.

In addition, the use of vortioxetine, like with all antidepressants, in the last trimester of pregnancy was associated with higher incidence of respiratory distress and pulmonary hypertension, cyanosis, apnea, seizures, temperature instability vomiting, hypoglycemia, hypotonia, hyperreflexia, tremor, irritability, constant crying and jitteriness, which required prolonged hospitalization, tube feeding and respiratory support.

The risk of the newborn to develop Persistent Pulmonary Hypertension of the Newborns (PPHN) is substantially higher compared to pregnant woman not on antidepressants. PPHN is associated with substantial neonatal morbidity and mortality.

Thus, the use of vortioxetine during the first trimester as well as throughout the pregnancy is not recommended.

Use during lactation

Vortioxetine is present in the milk of lactating rats. At this moment it is not known whether vortioxetine is secreted in the human breast milk. Due to its unknown effects on the newborn's normal growth and development breast feeding should be avoided.

Carcinogenesis

In mice, vortioxetine was not carcinogenic in both males or females at doses up to 24 times the maximum recommended human dose (MRHD). Treatment of rats with vortioxetine at doses up to 120mg/kg/day (58 times the MRHD) had no effect on males or females fertility.

Avoid using vortioxetine in the following cases

- **Patients with known allergy to vortioxetine**
- **Concomitantly with MAOI**

Vortioxetine's drug interactions

Follows a list of vortioxetine's drug interactions

- **Triptants**: The concomitant use may increase the risk of serotonin syndrome.

- **TCA**: The concomitant use may increase the risk of serotonin syndrome.
- **Lithium:** The concomitant use may increase the risk of serotonin syndrome.
- **Tramadol:** The concomitant use may increase the risk of serotonin syndrome.
- **Fentanyl:** The concomitant use may increase the risk of serotonin syndrome.
- **Tryptophan supplements:** The concomitant use may increase the risk of serotonin syndrome.
- **St. John's Wort:** The concomitant use may increase the risk of serotonin syndrome.
- **MAOI:** The concomitant use may cause Serotonin syndrome. Patients must wait 21 days after the MAOI was stopped before initiating treatment with vilazodone. Wait 5-7 days after discontinuing vilazodone before starting a MAOI.

Warning for vortioxetine

- **Pregnancy**: **Risk category C**. Try to avoid use during pregnancy or breast feeding. Assessment of the risks versus benefits must be discussed with the patient.
- **Seizure risk**. Vortioxetine was not associated with increased seizure activity. However, patients with a history of seizure require caution when using vortioxetine, as well as patients with an increased predisposition to have seizures, such as brain damage, as well as alcohol abusers.
- **Vortioxetine may cause an increase in suicidal risk in young adults**. The use of antidepressants in this population must balance the risk of suicide with the clinical need. Careful monitoring of the patients clinical

worsening is necessary. Evaluation for suicidality should also involve the family and all other caregivers.
- **Activation of hypomania or mania** may occur in vortioxetine-treated bipolar patients. As vortioxetine may trigger mania in predisposed patients, it should be used cautiously in patients with a history of bipolar mood disorder
- **Serotonin syndrome** may develop with vortioxetine use. Serotonin syndrome symptoms may include agitation, dizziness, hallucinations, delirium, seizures and coma along with autonomic instability, which includes tachycardia, fluctuating blood pressure, flushing, hyperthermia, tremor, muscular rigidity, myoclonus, hyperreflexia and incoordination. The concomitant use of vortioxetine with MAOIs, triptans, TCAs, lithium, fentanyl, tramadol, tryptophan, buspirone and St. John's Wort may precipitate serotonin syndrome.
- **Renal impairment**: Vortioxetine does not require a lower dose in mild to moderate renal impairment.
- **Liver impairment**: Vortioxetine does not require lower dose in patients with liver impairment..
- **Alcohol:** Vortioxetine did not increased the impairment of mental or motor skills caused by alcohol. However, it is not recommended to use vortioxetine in conjunction of alcohol.
- **Withdrawal reaction.** Vortioxetine use may result in a withdrawal reaction, prevention of which requires a slow reduction of vortioxetine dose. The withdrawal symptoms of vortioxetine can develop as early as the second day of the drug's sudden discontinuation and may persist for several days.
- **MAOI:** Vortioxetine's combined use with a MAOI may be fatal. Vortioxetine requires **7 day** washout period before starting with a MAOI. A **3 week** washout period is needed

after the MAOI was stopped before starting with vortioxetine.
- ➢ **Weight**: Vortioxetine was not associated with weight gain.
- ➢ **Abnormal bleeding:** The use of vortioxetine and other SSRIs may be associated with increased risk of bleeding. The concomitant use of aspirin, NSAIDs and warfarin may add to this risk. Bleeding has ranged from ecchymosis, hematoma, epistaxis and petechiae to life-threatening hemorrhage.
- ➢ **Hyponatremias**: Patients treated with diuretics may be at a greater risk of developing hyponatremia.
- ➢ **Angle Closure Glaucoma:** The use of vortioxetine can cause mild pupillary dilatation which in susceptible patients may cause an episode of angle closure glaucoma.

Vortioxetine overdose

There is limited clinical experience regarding vortioxetine overdose. There are only several overdose cases with vortioxetine limited to patients who accidentally consumed up to a maximum of 40mg.

Ingestion of vortioxetine in the dose range of 40- 75mg was associated with:

- Nausea
- Dizziness
- Diarrhea
- Abdominal discomfort
- Pruritus
- Somnolence
- flushing

The effects of vortioxetine overdose are also dependent on whether it was ingested alone or as a combination with other drugs and or with alcohol. As a general rule, the bigger the amount of vortioxetine ingested, the worse the toxic effects and the higher the possibility for lethal results.

Vortioxetine lethal action in mono therapy overdose- Unknown

The concomitant use of vortioxetine with alcohol and with other central nervous depressants such as painkillers or benzodiazepines may result in death caused by respiratory depression. The possible fatalities are often the result of cardio-respiratory arrest and the metabolic acidosis and hypoxia which are associated with status epilepticus.

What to do in the case of vortioxetine overdose

In general, there is no antidote for vortioxetine overdose. Management is mainly supportive, aimed at maintaining respiration, pulse and blood pressure. In the event of a recent overdose with vortioxetine, a stomach washout with activated charcoal might help in the elimination of the un-absorbed drug and is done with a large bore oro-gastric tube with appropriate airway protection. The aim of the stomach lavage is to get rid of the drug leftovers.

In some ER departments, ipecac is also used in order to induce vomiting of the ingested toxin, however **induction of emesis is not recommended in semi-comatose and comatose patients**. Due to the large volume of distribution of vortioxetine, forced diuresis, dialysis hemo-perfusion and exchange transfusion are unlikely to be effective. Keeping open the patient's airway is compulsory, especially in semi - comatose individuals. The patient should be placed on his side in order to prevent aspiration of the vomitus back to the lungs. Suffocation due to vomit is the leading cause of death in vortioxetine overdose. Blood pressure and heart rate monitoring is very important. Fluid intake should be monitored with intra-venous infusion of saline, and urinary output should also be carefully monitored. In most cases, vortioxetine overdose, requires hospitalization of the patient for at least 24 hours for intense observation.

Reference for Vortioxetine

1 Boulenger JP, Loft H., Olsen CK. Efficacy and safety of vortioxetine 15 and 20mg/day: a randomized, double blind, placebo controlled , duloxetine- referenced study in the acute treatment of adult patients with major depressive disorder. Int Clin Psychopharmacol, 2014 May: 29(3): 138-149.

Suggested general reading

Psychopharmacology

Julien RM, Advokat C, Comaty JE. A primer of drug action. Worth Publishers 2011.

Leonard Lichtblau. Psychopharmacology Demystified. Delmare Cengage Learning. 2011.

Meyer JS, Quenzer LF. Psychopharmacology. Drugs, the brain and behavior. Sinauer Associates, Inc.2005.

Harvey RA, Champe PC. Lippincott's Illustrated Reviews, Pharmacology Lippincott Williams & Wilkins 2006.

Nestler EJ, Hyman SE, Malenka RC. Molecular Neuropharmacology. A foundation for clinical neuroscience.McGraw Hill Medical 2009.

Rang HP, Dale MM,Ritter JM, Moore PK. Pharmacology. Churchill Livingstone 2003.

Kalyna Z. Bezchlibnyk-Butler, J. Joel Jeffries. Clinical handbook of Psychotropic drugs. 14 edition, Hogrefe & Huber 2004.

PG Janicak, SR Marder, MN Pavuluri. Principles and Practice of Psychopharmacotherapy. Fifth edition. Lippincott Williams & Wilkins, 2011.

Traetment

1 Stahl SM. Stahl's Essential Psychopharmacology. Cambridge University Press 2008.

2 Stahl S.M. The prescriber Guide. Cambridge University Press. 2011.

3 Schatzberg AF, Nemeroff C B. Essentials of clinical psychopharmacology. American Psychiatric Publishing Inc. 2006.

4 Papakostas GI, Fava M. Pharmacotherapy for Depression and Treatment Resistant Depression. World Scientific 2010.

5 Stein DJ, Lerer B, Stahl SM. Essential Evidence based Psychopharmacology. Cambridge University Press. 2012.

5 Kennedy SH, Gorwood P. Successful Management of Major Depressive Disorder. Evolving Medicine, Ltd 2012.

6 Stern TA, Fricchione GL, Cassem NH, Jellinek MS, Rosenbaum JF. Handbook of General Hospital Psychiatry. Saunders Elsevier 2010.

7 Kennedy SH, Lam RW, Nutt DJ, THase ME. Treating Depression Effectively.Martin Dunitz, informa healthcare, 2007.

Internet

www.dailymed.nlm.gov/dailymed/lookup

wwww.preskorn.com

www.medicine.iupui.edu/flockart

www.drugs.com

www.ingramcontent.com/pod-product-compliance
Lightning Source LLC
Chambersburg PA
CBHW051622170526
45167CB00001B/30